BALANCE YOGA

Chair Yoga for Parkinson's Disease and
other Movement Disorders

RHONA PARSONS, E-RYT500

The Balance Coach

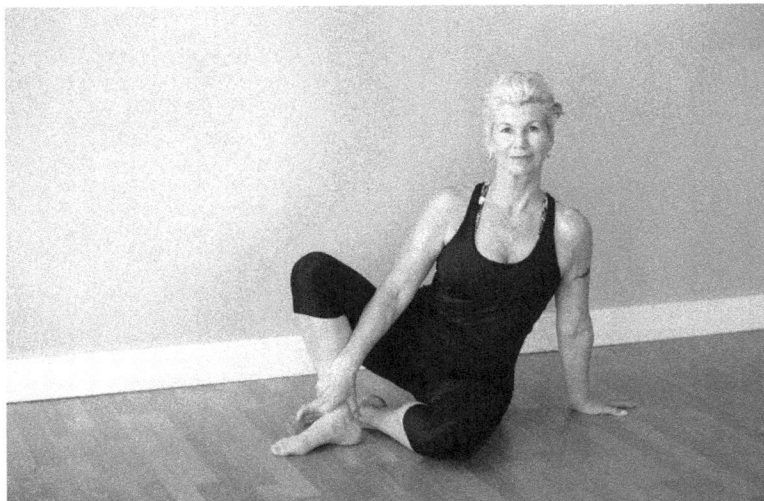

"Awareness is the beginning of change."

RUBY BLUE PUBLISHING

Published by Ruby Blue Publishing.

For information visit: www.rhonaparsons.com

Cover design by Shine Creative: www.shine-creative.ca

ISBN: 978-1-7753293-2-9

First edition: August 2019

To my clients, who have

wholeheartedly trusted me to help them prolong

the progression of PD...

I thank you for allowing me into your lives

to lead the way.

♥

CONTENTS

PREFACE

I have personally seen what happens when people with movement disorders embrace Yoga. Yoga helps create relaxation, which in turn helps control tremors in people with Parkinson's Disease (commonly known as PD). It activates affected muscle groups and can be a steady reminder of where your body should be and how it should move. I see the changes in my participants from when they first come into class to when they leave.

Since 2005, I have had the privilege and honor to work with individuals who have PD. Twice a week I meet with an amazing and very active group (both men and women) at a local gym whose collaborative goal is to keep prolonging the progression of the disease, reduce the symptoms, and restore function through exercise, yoga, and stretching. I have seen firsthand how these three disciplines have helped each one of them immensely with improvement in their balance, strength, flexibility, and mobility.

In 2013 I had the opportunity to travel to Arizona, USA, and spend a weekend with Dr. Becky Farley, the founder of PWR!, Parkinson Wellness Recovery, learning techniques, stretches, and exercises that Becky had researched to help improve quality of life for those with PD. It was a great weekend of learning and networking.

From 2012 to 2017, I was honored to organize the annual Parkinson Superwalk here in our town of 40,000 people and was amazed each year at the generosity of the community. Combining the walk and a silent auction, we raised a substantial amount of money for research; we are always hoping that a cure will be found sometime soon.

In 2005, a pilot study conducted at Cornell University placed 15 people with PD in 10 weeklong yoga programs, after which participants reported less trunk stiffness, better sleep, and a general feeling of well-being.

Yoga isn't a cure for Parkinson's Disease, but it can always help you come back to your center, balancing your body, mind, and emotions, bringing inner peace and happiness.

"Acceptance doesn't mean resignation…

It means to understand that something

is what it is and there's got to be a way through it."

Michael J. Fox

HOW YOGA HAS HELPED ME

Yoga has helped me in so many ways since being diagnosed with Parkinson's Disease (PD) in 2007. It has helped me on so many levels; physically, emotionally, and with my flexibility.

When I talk about Yoga helping me physically, with Parkinson, I experience the slowness of the muscles and movement, and I need to keep moving. The experience you get with Yoga helps you to keep moving all those muscles that you don't use regularly.

On an emotional level, you deal with issues such as grieving, issues such as stress and anxiety, and with yoga, you learn to breathe in a different way to what you usually do. My breath is quite often very shallow from the stress and anxiety that I experience daily. With Yoga, I breathe deeply and bring my body and mind back to a normal state of balance. This state reduces the symptoms of anxiety, stress, etc.

I meditate regularly, and Yoga helps with calming the mind and keeping me present. A lot is going on, especially when you are first diagnosed with Parkinson; you need to learn so many things, and it can be very overwhelming. Yoga helps with being overwhelmed by teaching how to calm the mind and find peace within yourself. I have learned a lot about mindfulness.

The beauty of Yoga is that you can do it anywhere; you can take your mat with you where ever you go. When I travel, I always have my mat with me. Yoga is the first thing I do in the morning as it helps with setting the intention for the day.

Rhona Parsons has helped me with my Yoga practice. She has been with me along my journey and has helped me to learn how to stretch and hold the poses, and giving me that little extra stretch when needed.

Yoga has helped me process all the changes that have happened in the past few years. Changes do happen, and we have to find ways to embrace the changes, along with all the other changes that happen with aging, with family, and with other incidents that happen in our lives. You don't need to be scared of Parkinson. If you practice Yoga, it will help you keep your confidence in pursuing the best you can be and changing your life where it still gives you that sense of satisfaction.

If you can, get down onto your mat and sit for a few minutes and do whatever comes to your mind, I promise you it will boost your mood. Yoga connects my body to my mind; it's what we all need to do in our busy lives, whether you have Parkinson's or not, it's what we all need to. Yoga is a very important part of my life. Bring it into your life, too; your body will thank you.

Jose Janssen., Armstrong, BC

A LOVE LETTER FROM PARKINSON

Dear Laura,

My name is Idiopathic Parkinson, and it's my time to thank you for your body that I now use as my vessel to progress and wreak havoc for all your years to come.

I've been watching you closely since I joined you, your husband, your family, and friends in February 2014, and I want to tell you that " I love you."

I reared my ugly head one hot, beautiful day in the Dominican Republic by making sure you or someone would notice I was forcing you to bend at the elbow on your right arm. Then, when no one noticed, quick enough for me, I made the arm stop swinging. Aha! Finally I was noticed, but you shrugged me off.

Well, you needed to know that I wasn't going anywhere. I just hung around, waiting patiently until a stressful event came into your life, a common way for me to introduce myself stronger, and sure enough, that event arrived. Your husband was diagnosed with bladder cancer and then told he could not have surgery to remove it because it was discovered he also needed a pacemaker. Bam! Perfect event!

I felt bad about my timing. However, it was my time to get you to take me seriously, so I gave you a right-hand tremor. Oh boy! How I enjoyed watching you spin; researching Google, trying to self-diagnose yourself for hours turning into days, but then, you all do.

That October you left to spend another hot winter in the Dominican Republic. I wasn't letting up on the tremor, so you decided to find two top Neurologists in Santo Domingo who could provide you with their opinions.

After many hours of research, you found your Neurologists, Dr. Santoni, and Dr. Ruiz, who both trained in England. Both are top in their field. Both came to the same conclusion; Me! Parkinson's!

Dr. Santoni was the first to tell you I was living in you. Watching your husband's head droop on the Doctor's desk while weeping, was by far the most intimate emotional moment I've shared with you.

I held your hand while you fell down a rabbit hole and couldn't claw yourself out. Day after day crying and asking, "Why? Why me at the age of 55?" Depression and denial took over, while I decided to add rigidity in your right shoulder to accompany the tremor in your right arm. Perfect combination. No right arm swing, shoulder rigidity, and tremor. Three of the cardinal signs that I have arrived.

You didn't snap out of it for weeks. I was starting to think you were not going to allow me to progress. You were scaring me, and I don't scare easily.

You decided to start a list titled *"What I hate most about Me, Parkinson's"*:

1. The unrelenting progression of symptoms. The thought that no matter what I do I will get worse with time because there's no cure

2. Constantly hiding my tremor by wearing pockets to hide it in

3. My fear I won't be able to take care of myself

4. My anger towards people who don't care to understand the severity of Parkinson's and its effect on our lives

5. Taking more meds than any human body can/should tolerate

6. Having to take meds for side effects caused by other meds and not by the disease itself

7. Being told we can live a normal life span but not realizing our years are filled with challenges and pain. Quantity is nothing without quality

8. The obligation to feel thankful for all the above because "I won't die due to Parkinson's, but my spirit may."

So, I pondered on all of the above and here's why "I love you":

1. You finally stopped wallowing in self-pity, stood up and decided to take me on, chanting your battle cry every morning in the mirror, "Bring it on!"

2. You're proactive in slowing me down by searching out what works best to delay my progression. Exercise! Good, old-fashioned exercise is the answer, and meds, as you need them.

3. Your daily relentless power walking of 8 kilometers a day. Joining two Parkinson's workout programs at a Gym that has programs specifically for me; boxing and circuit training taught by compassionate individuals who truly care about you; who truly want me to stick around longer by slowing me down, way down.

So I'll close my "love letter" to you by saying you are one tough competitor! You never let me down by allowing a depression in or giving up on me. You have learned to accept me, and by doing so, you adapted to our new life together. I Thank You.

Love Parkinson

Written by Laura Wilson, Vernon, BC

INTRODUCTION

This flowing Balance Yoga practice has been put together for anyone who has a movement disorder or for those of you who have been injured and needs a safe way to begin rehabilitation.

The book is also a great reference book for teachers who work with clients needing a safe, straightforward yoga practice.

If you are someone who has never exercised before, has been injured, has heart disease, PD, or another neurodegenerative disease, you have probably been told at some point or another by your neurologist/physiotherapist that you need to exercise.

If you think you are too old to start exercising, I want to tell you that **any age is the right age to exercise!** I know you probably don't want to read this, but I strongly urge you to start because it will make a difference for you.

Even if we take the disease or injury out of the equation, you still have a heart that needs to stay healthy, blood pressure, and cholesterol levels that need to stay in healthy levels. You may have osteoporosis; arthritis etc…the list is endless!

It is important to exercise because our body is meant to move; it has been created to move. We have all these joints in our body that make us move. We are not meant to be sitting for hours in a day; sitting on the couch, sitting behind the wheel of a car; we are meant to move.

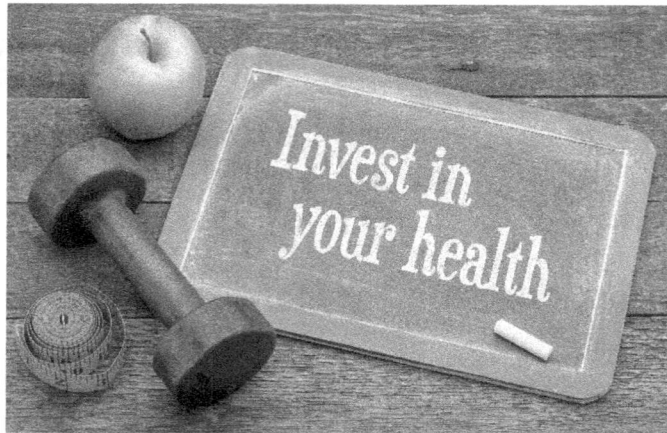

What do you like to do as a physical activity? Your pick is the first ingredient to success. If you begin something that you don't enjoy, you will only last a little while before you stop. What did you do for physical activity as a child that you loved? Memories are always a great place to look back on for ideas on what you like to do today.

Write it here:

_____

_____

Here are some examples of different ways to exercise broken down into categories. The word 'weight-bearing' means when your body works against the forces of gravity, and these are some of the best types of exercises to do. Pick all the activities that interest you:

LOW IMPACT WEIGHT-BEARING EXERCISES

- Low Impact Aerobics (cardio – low intensity)
- Walking
- Treadmill walking
- Stationary bicycle riding
- Elliptical training
- Swimming

HIGH IMPACT WEIGHT-BEARING EXERCISES

- Dancing
- Hiking
- Pickleball
- Tennis
- Cycling
- Ballet
- Jazz Dancing
- Boxing

<u>MUSCLE STRENGTHENING EXERCISES</u>

- Weightlifting
- Using weight machines
- TRX (bodyweight) straps
- TheraBands and exercise tubing

<u>CORE, FLEXIBILITY AND BALANCE EXERCISES</u>

- Yoga
- Pilates
- Core-specific classes
- Ballet

As you can see, there are a variety of things to do to keep your heart healthy, your bones strong, and to keep the spring in your step. You don't have to join the gym to lift weights or a dance class to dance if you don't like being in a group atmosphere.

I know my group of participants in the PD class enjoy working out with each other. They are very supportive of one another, and they have great conversations on different topics; symptoms they might be experiencing, their neurologists, research they have read about, etc.

The one thing the group loves to participate in is the yoga stretching that we do at the end of class. The stretching that we do is called Static Stretching, a holding stretch. We want to put our body into a specific position that will work on releasing tightness and lengthen our muscles. Some of the yoga poses in this book are static stretches. When your body relaxes into the stretch, you can stay there for as long as it feels good.

Other poses that we do (in the book) are Dynamic stretches. This form of stretching is stretching with movement, and it will get your body prepared for your yoga practice.

Performing dynamic movements as a warm-up before the work has many benefits; it will increase blood flow to the body, as your body gets warmer, your movements will get bigger, and you will begin to feel more energized, to name a few.

Sometimes when poses are held (static) for too long by a person with PD, he/she can experience tremors. For this reason, we don't hold poses for very long in each movement sequence in this practice.

<u>YOGA</u>

Yoga is an old discipline from India that has been around for about five thousand years. It is a system that is both spiritual and physical and helps us with self-discovery. The system is made up of 8 limbs or pathways that take us to this realization. One of these limbs is known as ASANA. In Sanskrit, asana means 'posture' or 'pose' and is the physical portion of Yoga.

There are many different styles of asana, but the one that is known by most is Hatha Yoga. This style of asana connects breath with movement, keeping you in the present moment while you are moving through the postures. It is also the path toward creating a balance of opposites. The word Hatha is broken down to translate as Ha = sun and tha = moon. When you are in a posture, you are looking to find the balance between the effort and ease of the pose.

There are many benefits to a Hatha Yoga practice:

- The Increase of strength and flexibility
- Improvement of balance and core strength
- Development of mindfulness
- Relief of chronic pain
- Reduction in anxiety and depression
- Improvement of sleep and quality of life

I am sure by now that you are starting to understand why you must move. Let's get started!

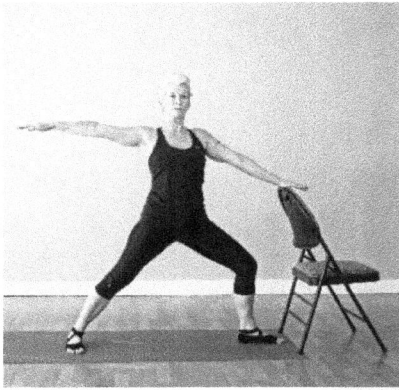

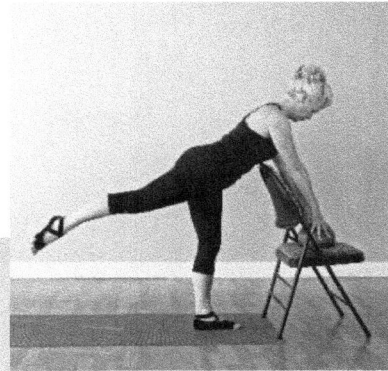

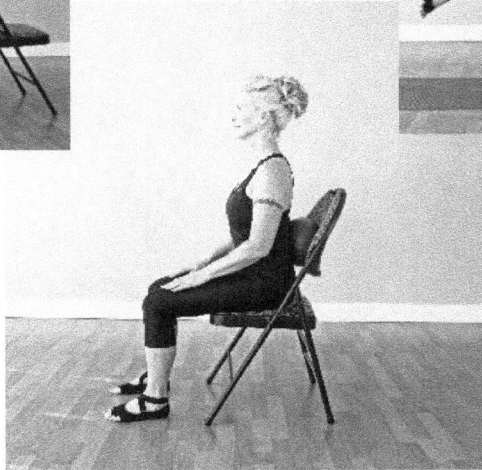

"The most important pieces of equipment you need for doing yoga are your body and your mind."

Rodney Yee

CHAPTER 1

GUIDELINES FOR A SAFE & EFFECTIVE YOGA PRACTICE

In this yoga workout, a chair is used for balance, but this practice can easily be done without the use of the chair if it's not needed.

1. **Practice on an empty stomach.**

    Wait at least 1 hour after eating.

    (For the PD client, you may want to wait until after you have taken the first bout of medication...for the instructor, scheduling your class around this time will help the client greatly).

2. **Practice regularly.**

    Even 10 minutes daily. Yoga is a *way of life,* not just an exercise program, and can help you get back in balance emotionally and physically. It is not a cure for PD, but it can bring you gently back to yourself every time.

3. **Always breathe normally in Yoga.**

    In yoga, movement follows the breath. We exhale into a pose and inhale coming out of the pose, allowing the body to flow with the wave of our breathing. Breathe fully and follow your rhythm of breathing. If your breath is strained, your body is likely to be too.

4.   **With every pose always remind yourself of the four basics:**

- Create balance at the base
- Be well-grounded
- Be mindful of the extension and contraction as you stretch
- Breathe as you hold the poses.

5.   **Never hurry.**

Go slowly into and out of each pose. Take 5-10 seconds to go into and come out of each posture. This will:

- Make each pose more beneficial
- Reduce the number of repetitions needed for optimum results
- Eliminate all chance of injury.

Remember the quality of movement is better than the quantity.

6.   **Never force a pose.**

Overworking rigid and tight muscles can cause spasms (cramps) but stretching too much (too far) can tear soft tissue.

Take your time and never extend to pain. Pause at any time you need to rest and stop any time you feel dizzy. Breathe.

7. **Holding postures once you have gone as far as you can into a pose.**

   Flowing (moving) in and out of poses, rather than holding, is more beneficial to people with PD because holding a pose can trigger involuntary muscle contraction, spasms, and overheating. Moving gently and allowing for resting breaths brings a healthy approach on and off the mat/chair.

8. **Don't judge. Just Notice. Rest comfortably in the present.**

9. **Never compare yourself to others; not even yourself.**

   Each day is different, and Yoga always focuses our attention on the present moment. Yoga is gently progressive meaning that you will progress at the pace that is right for you. So that you don't hurt yourself, only stretch to where it feels right for you.

10. **Rest between poses.**

    Yoga is gentle. Yoga is meditative. Yoga energizes as you breathe and relax.

Rest periods:

- Allow muscles a chance to gently return to their natural resting length after a delightful stretch
- Gives you a delicious moment to connect with yourself
- Invite in the sensation of pleasure that comes after slow stretching.

11. Don't get discouraged.

Somedays, your practice will be better than others. Give yourself a break. Always listen to your body and give it what it is asking for in that present moment. Know that tomorrow is another day.

12. Dress comfortably.

Some clothing can restrict movement, so make sure that you aren't wearing tight clothes, a belt, or anything else that doesn't allow your body to move freely.

CHAPTER 2

PROPS TO CONSIDER USING

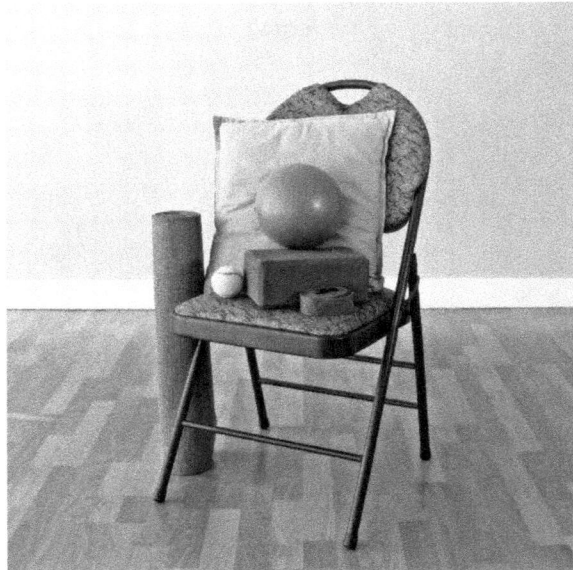

- A chair with a back, preferably with no armrests
- A yoga mat
- One or two yoga blocks
- A tennis ball or something softer
- A yoga strap - approx. 6 feet long
- A pliable ball (approx. 7-8 inches in diameter). Using a pliable ball behind the back when sitting helps you sit taller and helps create and encourage stronger core muscles.
- A rolled-up towel will work if a ball is not available.

CHAPTER 3

THE BREATH

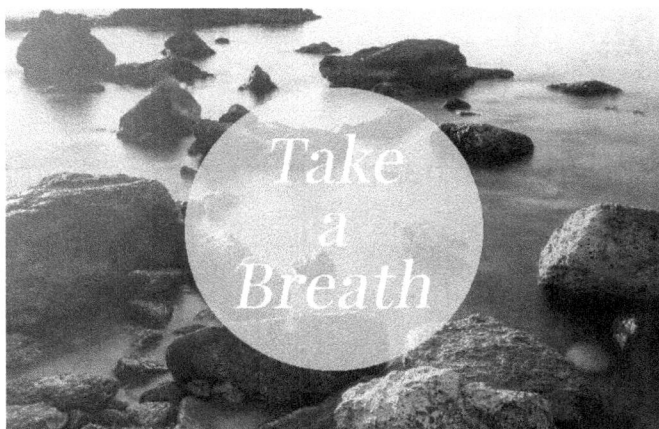

Breathing is one of our most vital functions in life.

Lowering your blood pressure, an increase in lung capacity and reduced anxiety are some of the benefits of practicing breathing.

For this yoga class, we combine three breathing (Pranayama) techniques:

1. **The Complete breath** is a 3-part breathing technique that brings about calmness, steadiness, quietness of the mind, and promotes relaxation.

2. Adding the **Ujjayi (Victorious) breath** (a whispering sound made at the base of the throat) to **The Complete breath**, the client begins to create a focus that helps him/her stay in the present moment. Ujjayi balances the inhalation with the exhalation and helps calm the nervous system. Both the inhalation and exhalations are through the nose.

3. LATERAL BREATHING. This technique teaches the client how to strengthen his/her core by focusing on contracting the abdominals.

THE COMPLETE BREATH

Sitting tall in the chair, place your hands on your thighs. Inhale slowly through the nose and breathe into your belly, gently pushing your belly out.

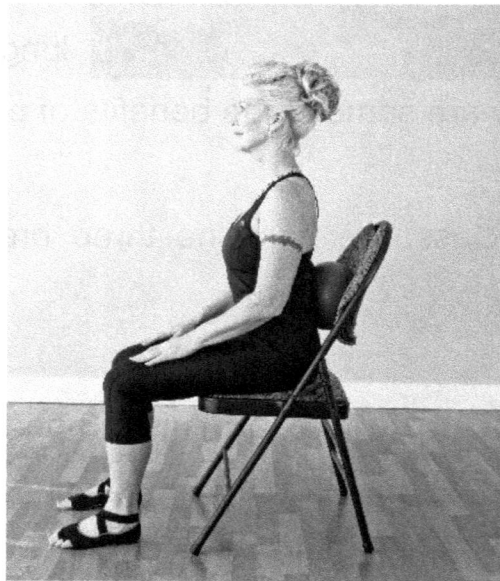

Exhale slowly through the nose and allow the belly to float towards the spine.

On the next inhale as the belly pushes outward, feel your ribcage expand and your upper chest rise.

Exhale and sense the belly pull in, the rib cage close and the chest fall. Repeat 4-6 times, breathing slowly and equally in and out.

Notice the calmness of your breath and mind.

In the Yoga tradition, we learn that the upper lungs feed our brain, head and upper limbs with prana (breath), the middle area of the lungs feed our torso with prana, and the lower area of the lungs feeds our lower limbs with prana.

> **Another way to stay focused is to listen to the mantra of the breath, SO HAM "I am that I am." As you breathe in hear the word "SO" and as you breathe out, the word "HAM".**

*MUDRAS (closure/seal)

Hand mudras are used in Yoga and can be used to direct the energy in the body to where we want it to go. Using certain mudras will help you perfect **The Complete breath** by connecting with and strengthening the entire area of the lungs.

Chin Mudra - Diaphragmatic Breathing

Touch the tips of the thumb and index finger together; other fingers straight. Place hands, palms down, on top of thighs with elbows directing outward; a slight pressure between the fingers and thumbs. Breathe easily for a few minutes feeling the rhythm of the breath and the movement of the diaphragm and lower ribs.

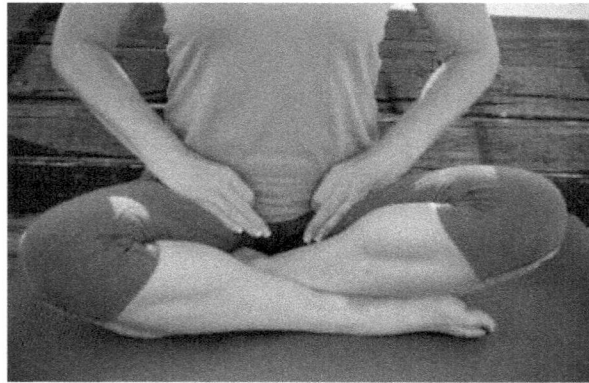

Chinmaya Mudra - Intercostal Breathing

Keeping the tips of the thumbs and index finger touching, curl remaining fingers into palms and place hands back down on thighs; palms down with the same slight pressure between fingers and thumbs. Breathe easily and bring focus to the flow of breath and the movement of the ribs around the middle of the chest.

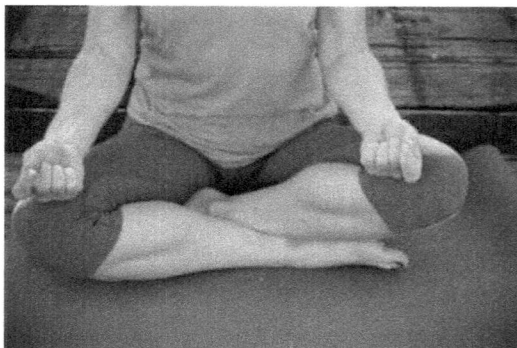

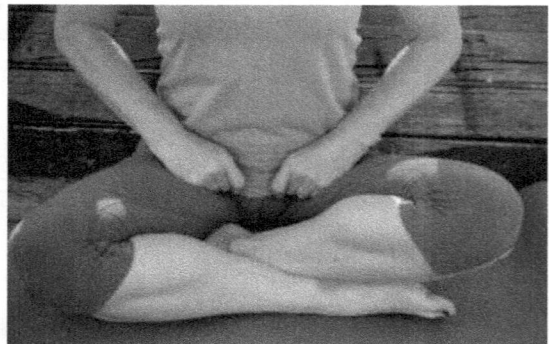

Ardhi Mudra - Clavicular Breathing

Open hands out and place thumbs across palms. Curl fingers over thumbs and place palms down on top of the thighs. Keep slight pressure on the fists and direct elbows outwards. Breathe easily concentrating on flow of breath and movement in the upper part of the ribcage.

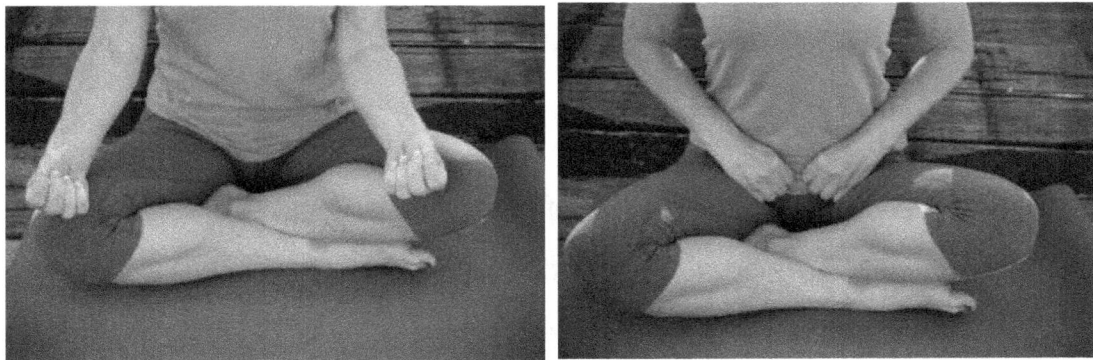

Brahma Mudra - Complete Breath

Turn **Ardhi Mudra** upwards and place hands at the naval. Focus on the flow of breath noticing that all three areas of the lungs are affected; first the lower area, then the middle and lastly the top of the lungs. Repeat the complete breath 8-10 times and then place hands back on thighs and relax.

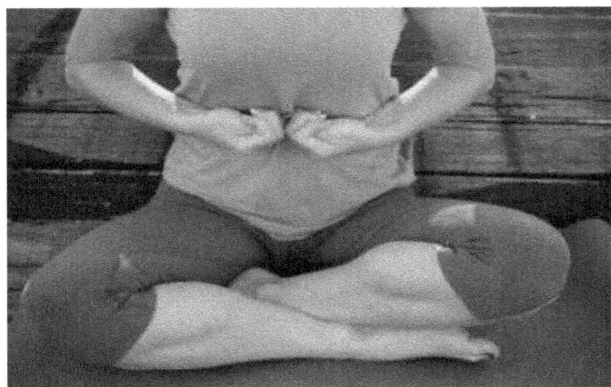

UJJAYI (Victorious) BREATH

Continuing with **The Complete breath**, and breathing in and out through the nose, begin to create a whispering sound at the back of the throat. This noise will help you focus and keep you in the present moment.

LATERAL BREATHING

Our core begins at the base of our neck and goes to the tops of our thighs. Strengthening the core not only helps us with balance but also promotes posture and lifts our chest giving us space to breathe.

When we pull our belly in towards the spine and up towards the ribcage, the belly doesn't expand when we inhale. Lateral breathing teaches us how to expand our ribcage sideways and into our back, still being able to get a full intake of air.

Let's Practice. Sit tall in the chair and pull your belly in towards the spine.

Keeping the belly pulled in, inhale and feel the breath going into the mid-chest, expanding the ribcage.

Exhale; start to actively pull your belly in towards your spine, contracting the abdominal muscles until the breath is out of the lungs.

Continue breathing this way. With each breath you take in, you will notice your core getting tighter and your ribcage becoming more mobile as the ribs can expand more. This separating develops length and strength through the torso and allows the lungs to expand more, bringing more oxygen into the body.

"When the breath wanders the mind is also unsteady, but when the breath is still, so is the mind still."

Hatha Yoga Pradipika

You have probably come to realize that sitting tall helps create great posture allowing you to breathe fully into the lungs enabling you to breathe easier.

The benefits of quality breathing:

- Lowers anxiety
- Decreases stress levels
- Calms the body
- Relieves chronic pain
- Allows you to rest longer and easier.

Breathe through it,
and release anything
that does not serve you

CHAPTER 4

THE FEET

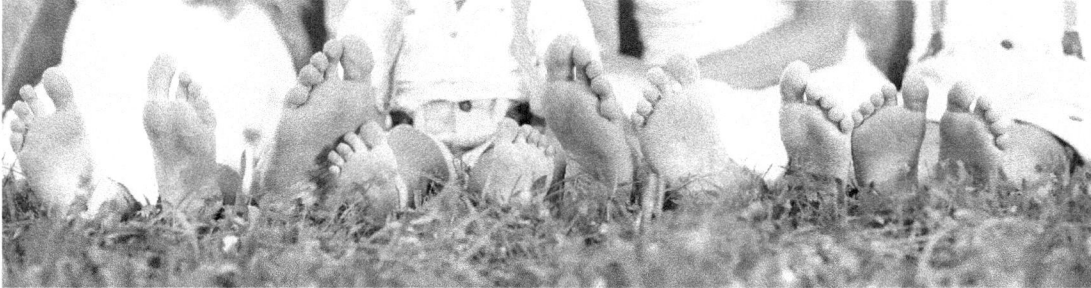

Our feet are our foundation and connection to the earth, and we need to look after them. When we have the chance to stretch our toes and our feet, we need to take the time to do it.

Relaxing the feet and stretching your toes apart, creating space between them, will improve tightness and aches and pains that you might be experiencing. Moving your toes back and forth helps keep the front arch in your feet mobile, which in turn will help you with balance, posture, and stability when you walk.

The feet are full of nerve endings that connect to other parts of our bodies. Rolling our feet on top of a small ball will "wake up" the nerve endings and increase the mobility and flexibility in the feet. It can increase the circulation and decrease any aches or pains we are experiencing in our feet or any other part of our body.

BALL ROLLING

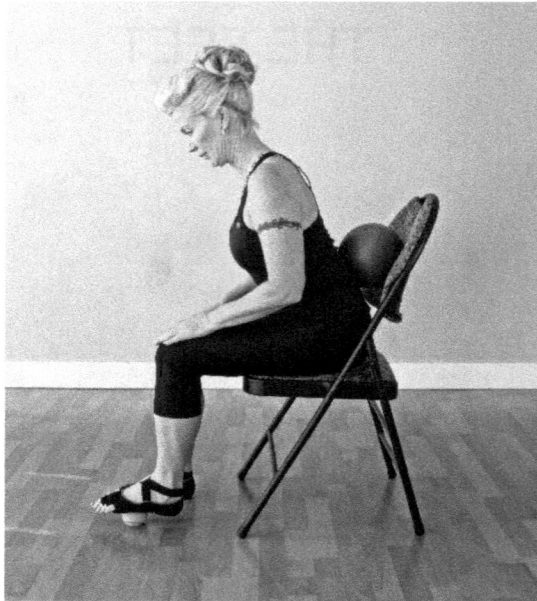

Sit tall with the ball behind your back and lean forward from the hips, creating a long spine. Place a tennis ball (or a softer ball) under one foot and begin to roll the ball back and forth from heel to toes.

When you find a "hurt so good" spot, stop rolling and press down with your foot, leaning slightly forward to enhance the pressure and to release the tension. Hold as long as you want.   Continue rolling the foot for 2-3 minutes. Notice how your ankles feel – not so tight and rigid?

Take your foot off the ball and place it on the floor. Feel the floor with your entire foot and notice any tingling sensations you are feeling (this is a good thing!). Repeat the exercise with your other foot.

THE ANKLE ALPHABET

abcdefghijklmn
opqrstuvwxyz

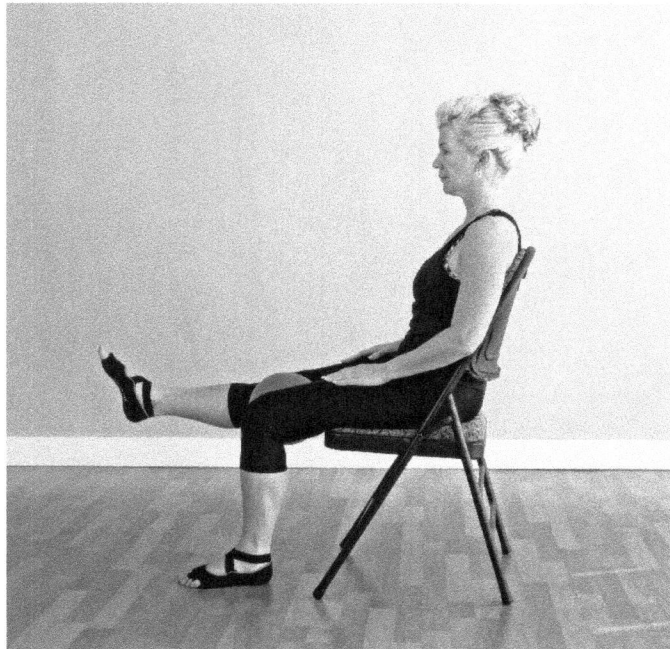

Sit tall again, lean back into the chair and place the ball between your legs, just above your knees. Straighten one leg.
Moving from your ankle, draw the alphabet (lower case letters) with your foot. Try to keep your leg still.

Repeat the alphabet with the other leg.

CHAPTER 5

POSTURE

What is good posture? Posture is the position in which you hold your body upright against gravity while standing, sitting, or lying down.

Good posture:

- Helps us breathe easier
- Keeps our bones and joints in correct alignment so that our muscles can move more effectively
- Reduces stress on our ligaments
- Helps prevent backache and muscle pain
- Prevents body fatigue (the body can move more efficiently, therefore, not using more energy for everyday movement)
- Helps avoid falling
- Strengthens our back and opens our chest.

The words **Power Up posture** will now be used as a cue to sit up tall. The purpose of this cue is to bring awareness of your posture against gravity. You will be focusing on sitting up tall, opening your chest (pulling your shoulders back) and pulling the belly in towards the spine. This posture fights against gravity and aids in stretching and strengthening the torso equally.

POWER UP POSTURE- SEATED

NEUTRAL SPINE

- Place feet flat on the floor and knees in line with feet, hip-distance apart. Sit tall on Sits Bones (see diagram below)

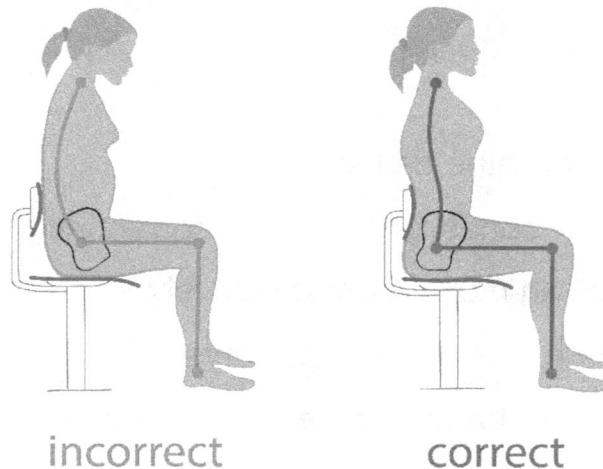

incorrect   correct

- Pull the belly in towards the spine and up towards the ribcage, creating space between the hips and ribs. Lift the chest, pull the shoulder blades back and down, spreading them wide across the ribcage, and bring the ears in alignment with the center of shoulders.

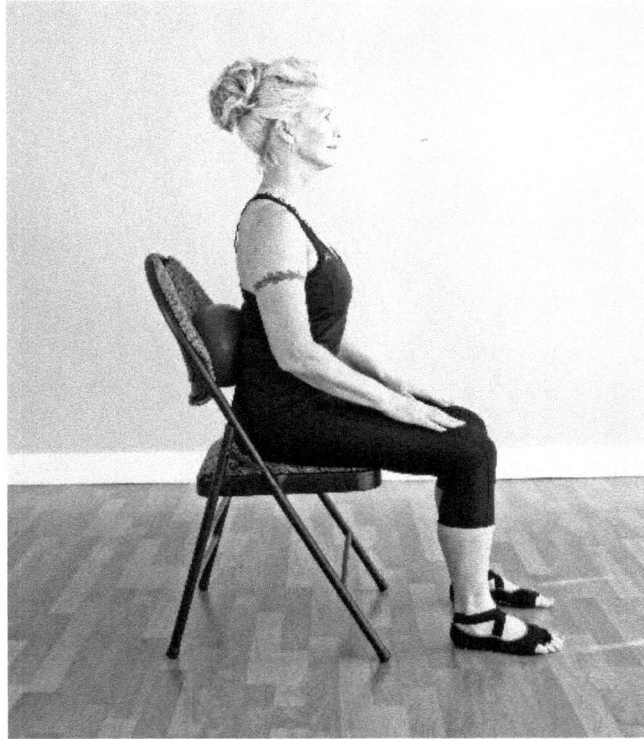

Side view alignment:

An invisible line should run through the ear, shoulder, and the hip. The knees stack over the ankles, and the legs should be hip-width apart.

"A moving body will never stiffen."

Joseph Pilates

CHAPTER 6

WARMING THE BODY

<u>NECK STRETCHES</u>

1. Power Up posture against the ball; spine long.

Exhale; pull belly towards the spine;

Inhale

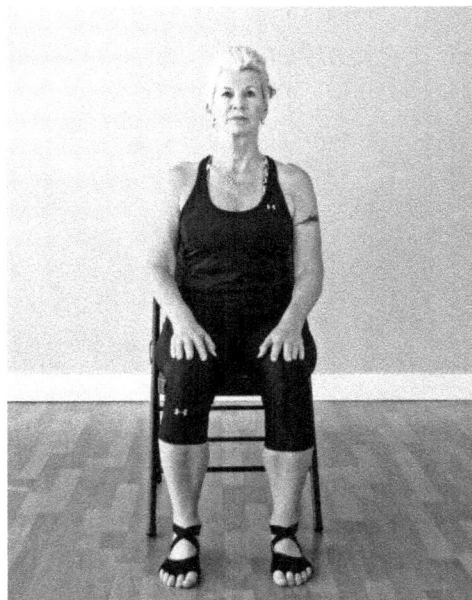

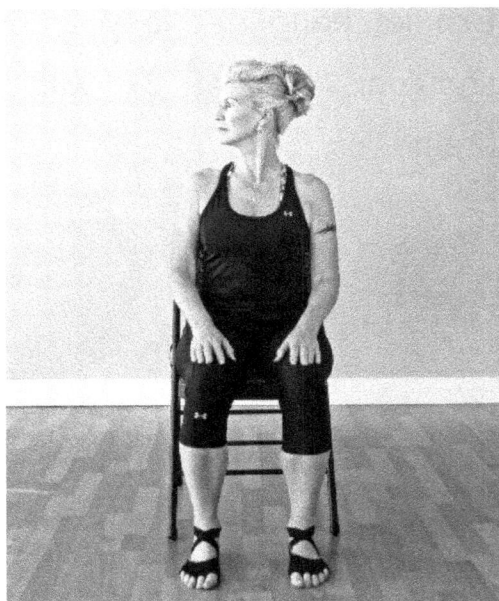

Exhale; turn your head to one side, only as far as it feels comfortable.

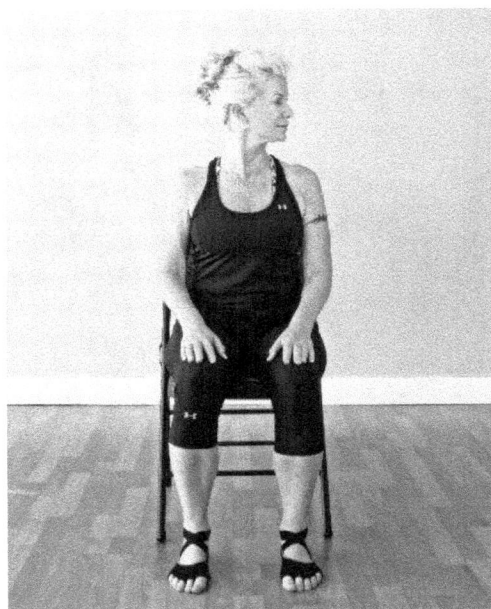

Inhale; bring the head to the center.

Exhale; turn head to the other side.

Repeat 3x each side with breath.

2. Exhale; gently tip one ear to shoulder

Inhale; bring your head back to the center

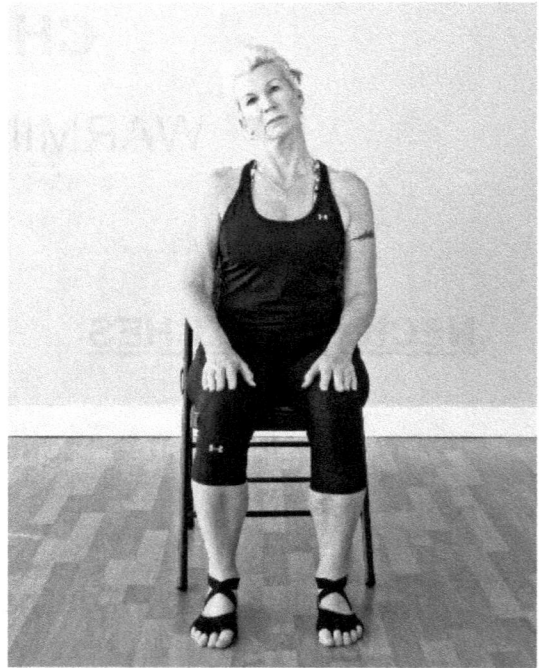

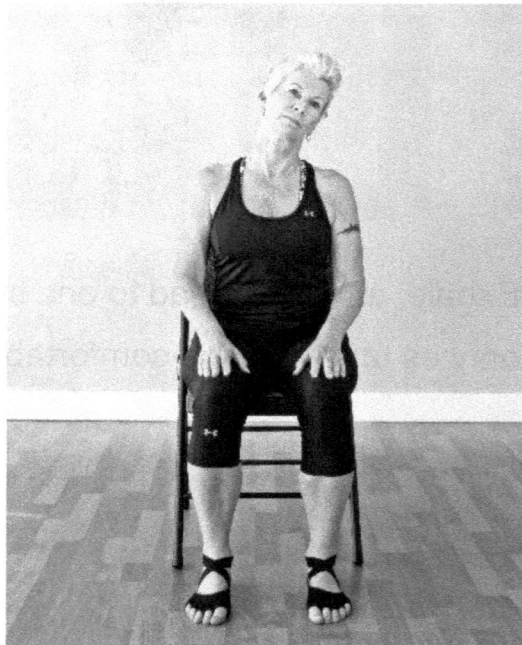

Exhale; bring ear to your other shoulder. Repeat 3x with the breath.

*"You cannot do yoga. Yoga is your natural state.
What you can do are yoga exercises, which may reveal to you
where you are resisting your natural state."*

Sharon Gannon

WRIST STRETCHES

Create the Power Up posture with the ball behind your back.

Grab right hand with the left hand and gently bend the hand down and up 3x. Hold down for 2-3 breaths

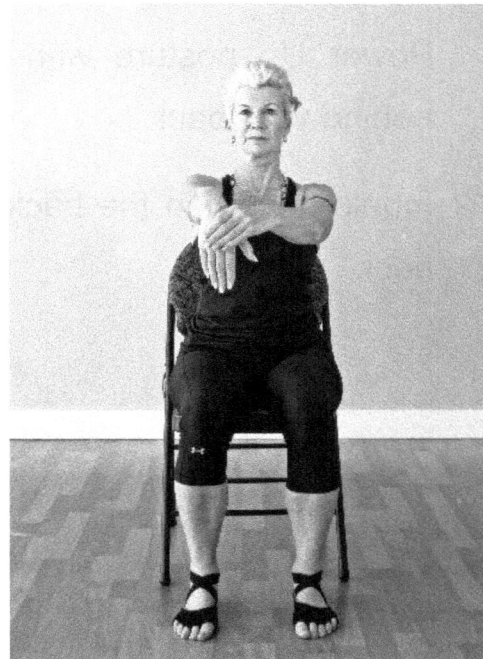

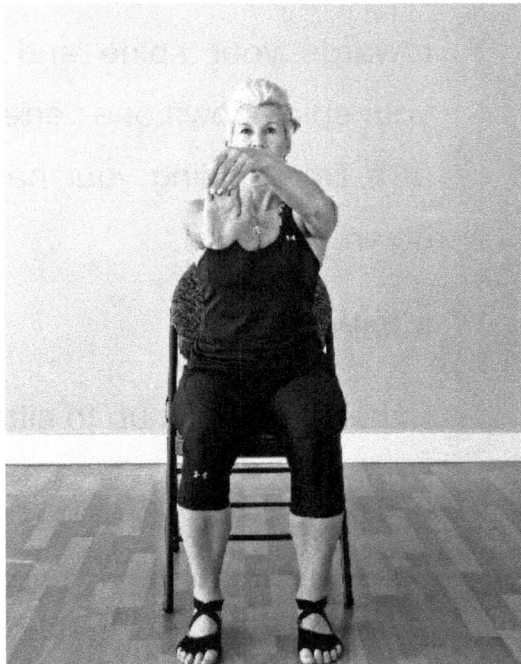

Lift hand upward at the wrist) and hold for a further 2-3 breaths, gently stretching forearms and wrists.

Repeat with the left hand.

ROLLDOWN

Power Up posture with the ball behind your back

Inhale; lengthen the back of your neck.

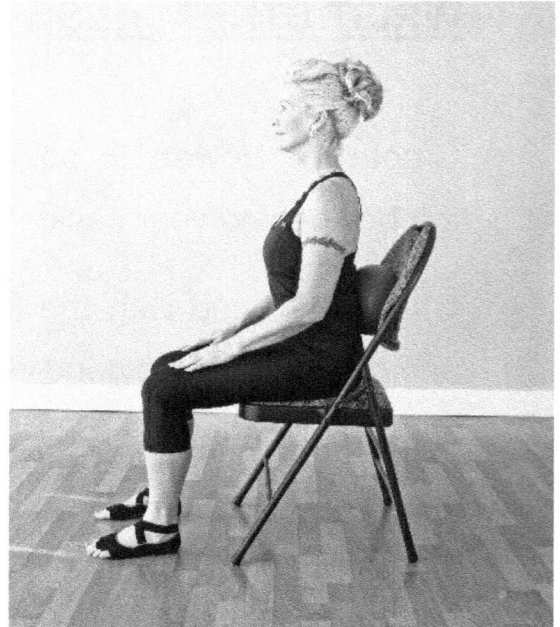

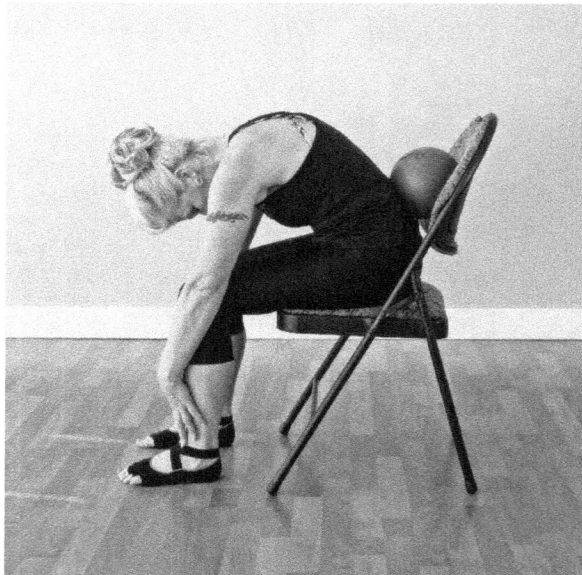

Exhale; pull your belly towards your spine and roll your spine down one vertebra at a time, sliding your hands down your legs.

Inhale;

Exhale; roll back up to sitting.
Repeat 3x

BENEFITS: To bring awareness and mobility to the spine.

PRECAUTION: High/low blood pressure: roll up and down very slowly

---

FORWARD BEND (Uttanasana)

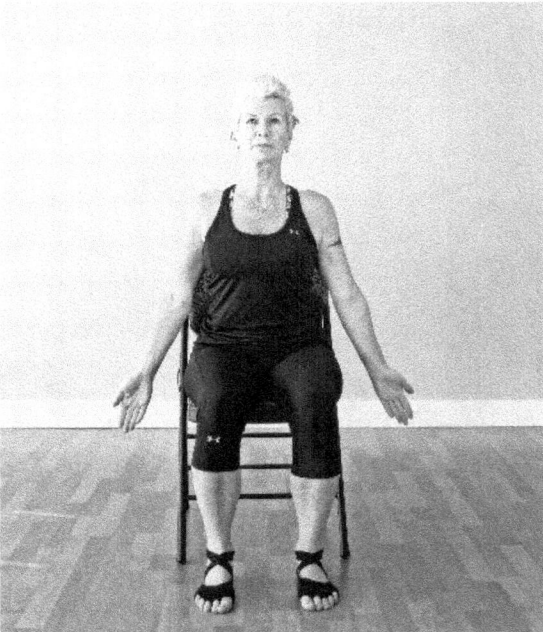

Power Up your posture with the ball behind your back, arms long and tight against your sides, palms facing forward.

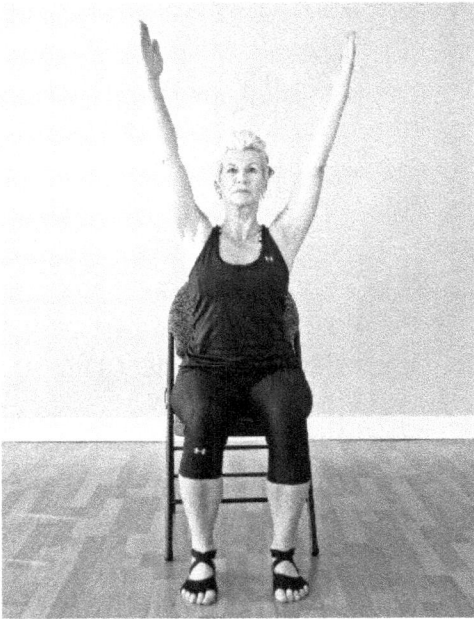

Inhale; reach arms up

Exhale; pull belly to spine and hinge

forward from hips, coming as low as it feels comfortable.

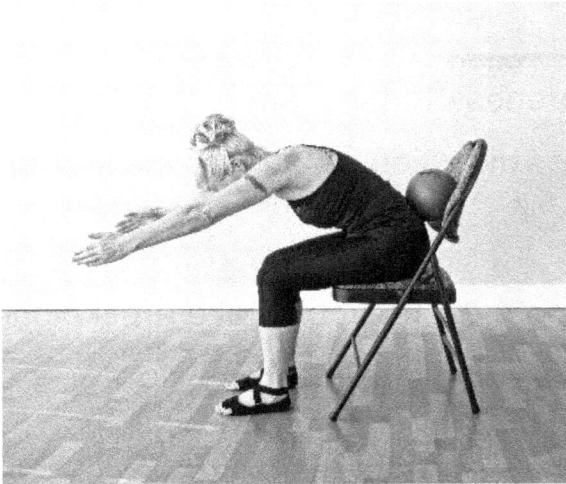

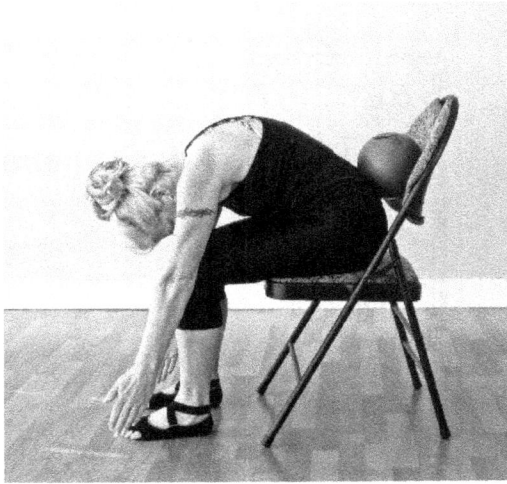

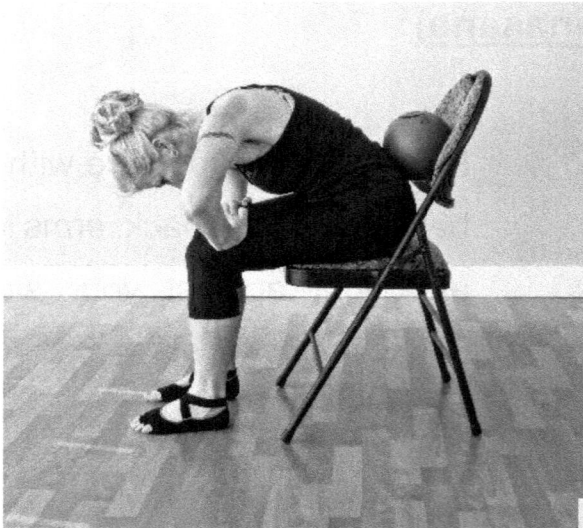

Inhale; place hands on thighs

Exhale; roll spine up one vertebra
at a time.

Repeat rolldown 3x

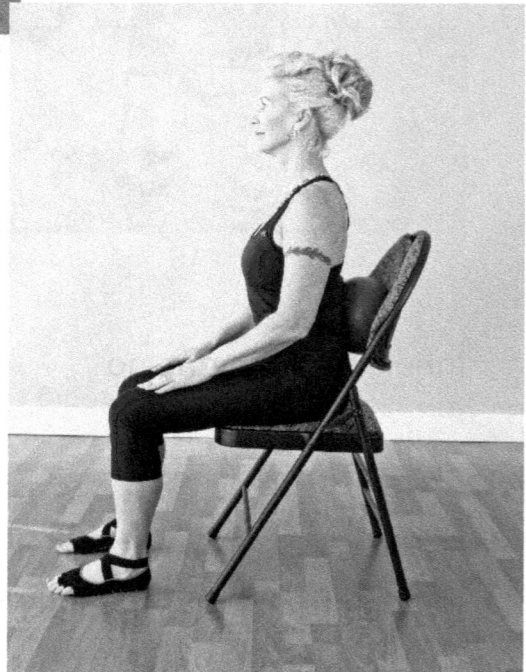

BENEFITS: Bringing awareness to hips, strengthening core, stretches low back, improves digestion, stimulates the liver and kidneys.

PRECAUTIONS: High blood pressure: don't take arms higher than shoulders. Low blood pressure: roll up very slowly

SHOULDER CIRCLES

Inhale; lift shoulders to ears

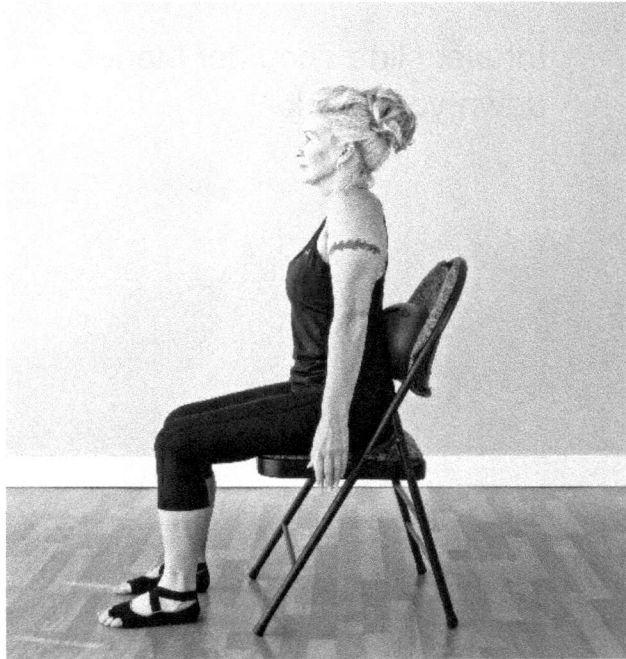

Exhale; start to roll
shoulders back

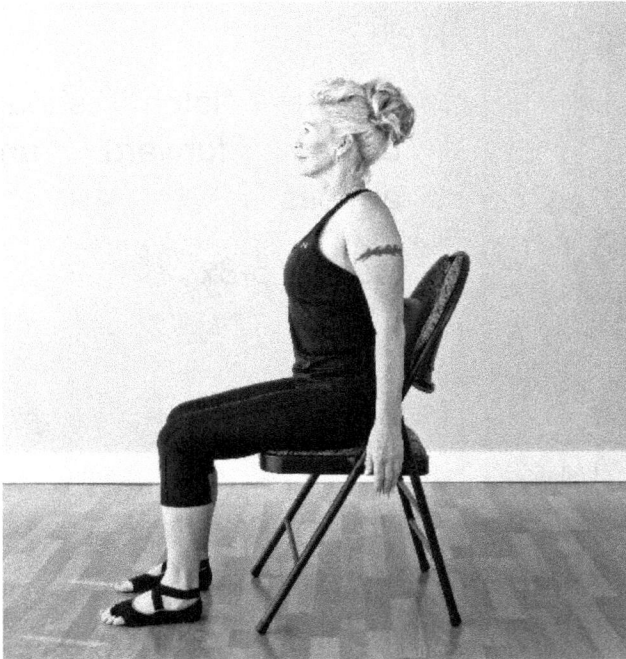

Inhale; slide shoulder blades down your back

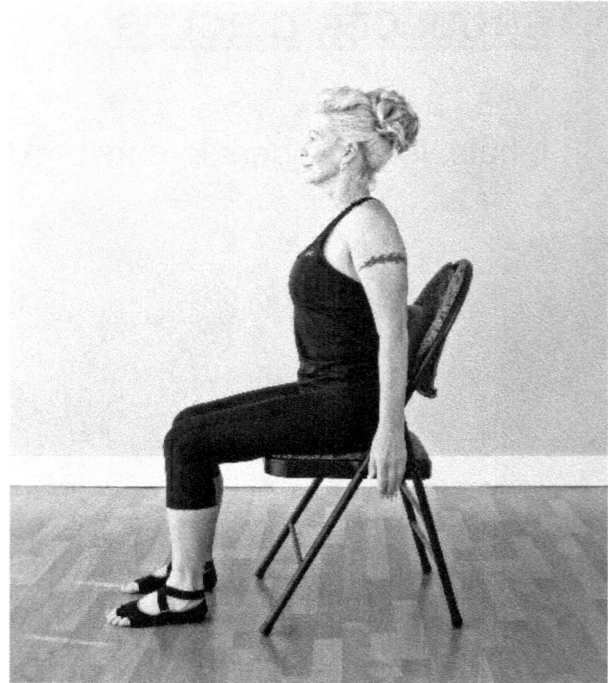

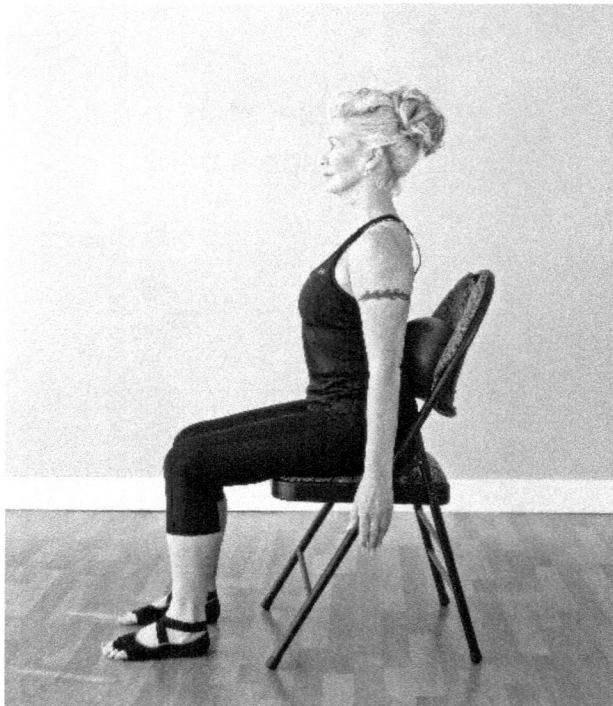

Exhale; "latch" shoulder blades forward under armpits.

Repeat 5-8x

BENEFITS: To increase shoulder blade mobility and flexibility; postural awareness, and increase lung capacity

<u>SIDE BEND</u>

Power Up posture with the ball behind the back, arms long and tight against your sides.

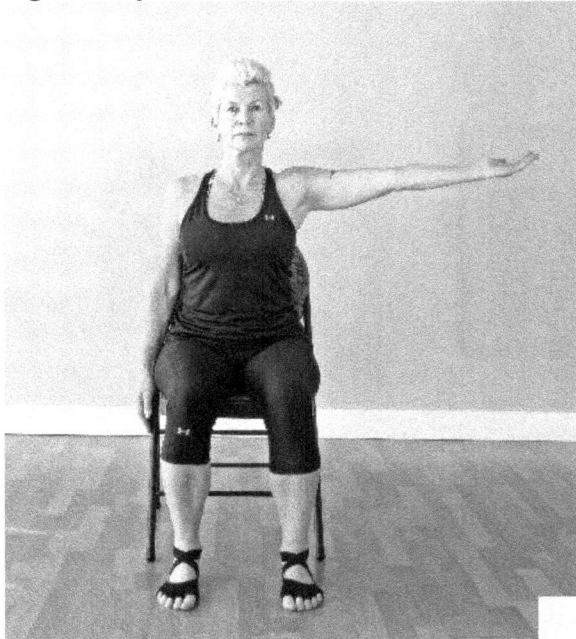

Inhale; reach left arm up to the height of your shoulders, palm up

Exhale; reach arm up and over, making sure your weight stays evenly under buttocks

Inhale; reach arm up

Exhale; come back and sit tall.

Repeat 3x on the same side before changing to the right arm.

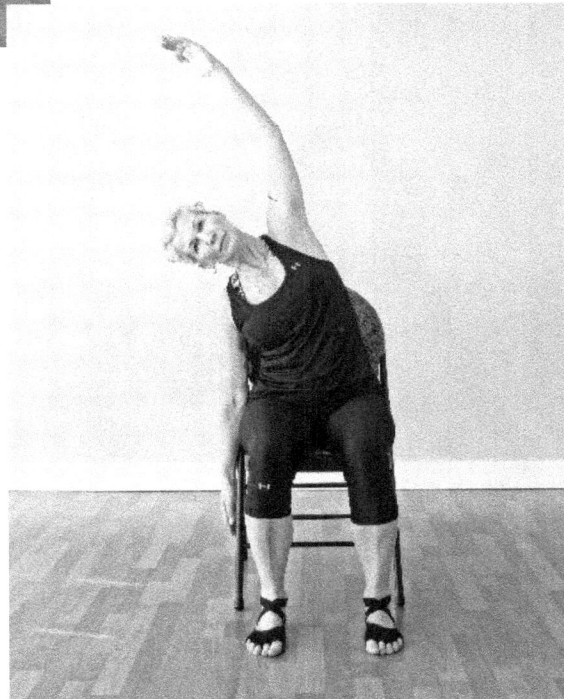

BENEFITS: To increase stretch on sides of body

ELBOW CIRCLES

Power Up posture with the ball behind back; place fingertips on shoulders. Inhale; sit tall

```
┌─────────────────────────────────┐
│ MODIFICATION: Place hands       │
│ on opposite shoulders if        │
│ unable to lift elbows           │
└─────────────────────────────────┘
```

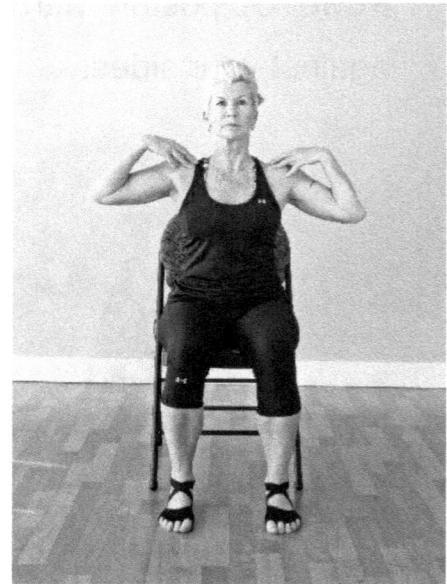

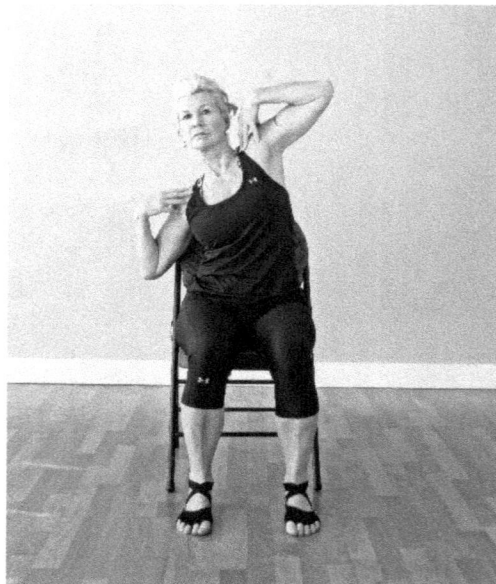

MODIFICATION: Place hands on opposite shoulders if unable to lift elbows

Exhale, pull belly to spine and rotate the body to the right, taking right elbow behind you. Inhale; back to the center

Exhale; pull belly to spine and rotate left.

Repeat 5x each side

BENEFITS: Increase mobility and flexibility in spine and waist

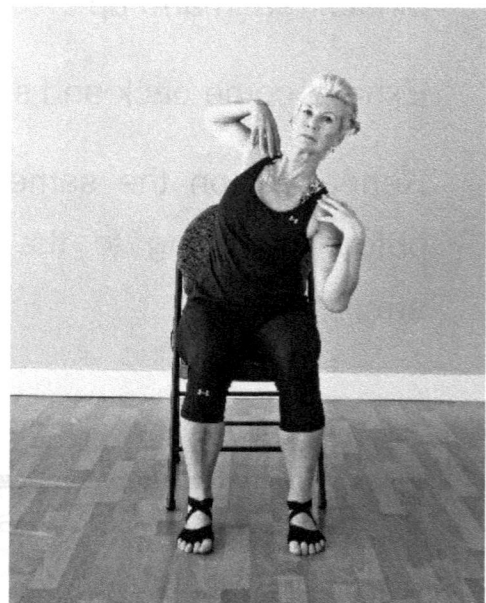

SEATED TWIST I

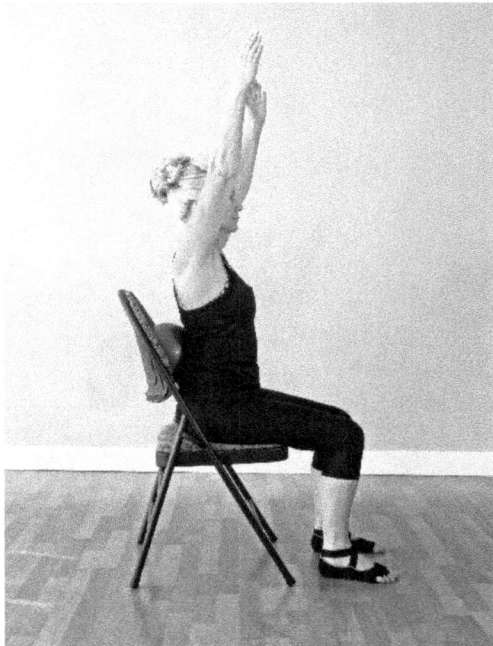

Power Up posture with the ball behind the back.

Inhale; bring arms up overhead

Exhale; pull belly to spine and keeping hips still, twist to the left, bringing arms down to the height of your shoulders; one arm back and one arm forward.

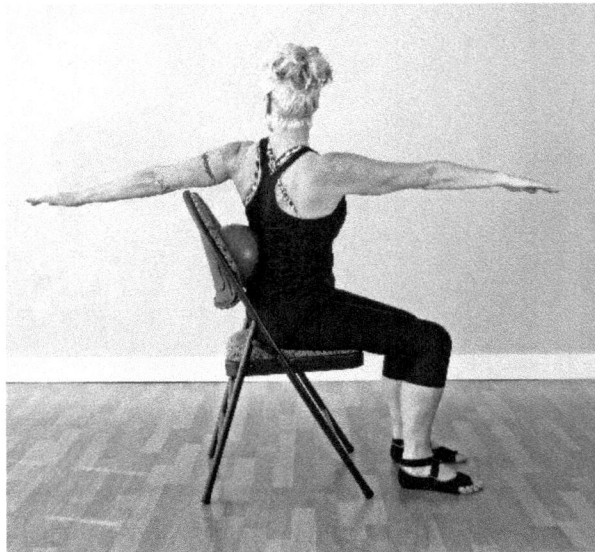

Inhale; breathe into ribs and come to the center

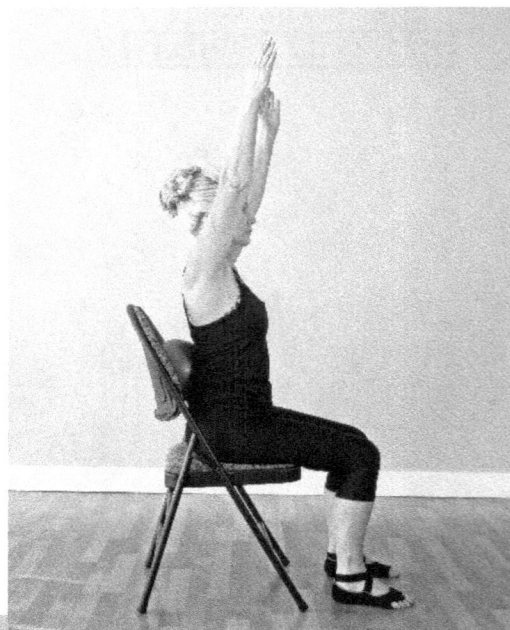

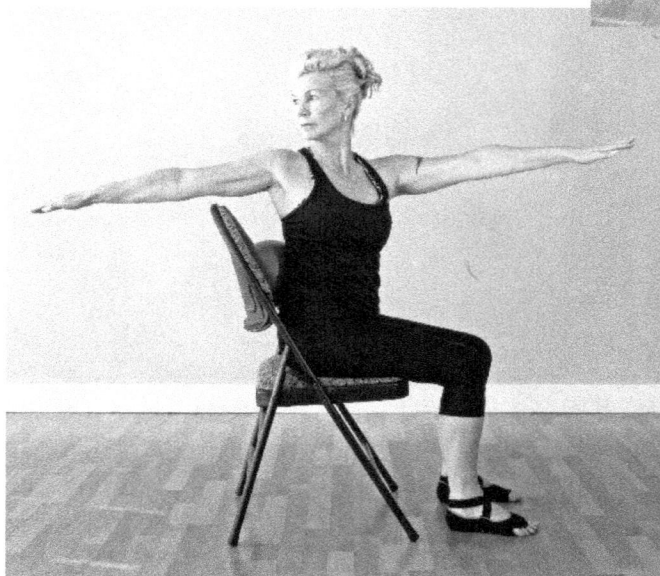

Exhale; repeat on the other side.

Repeat 3x each direction.

BENEFITS: Improves posture, increases lung capacity, flexibility and mobility in the spine and waist. Opens chest and shoulders.

PRECAUTION: Do not hold your breath, and only turn as far as it feels comfortable.

EXECUTIVE STRETCH:

Power Up your posture with the ball behind your back, hands behind head, making your head very heavy in your hands.

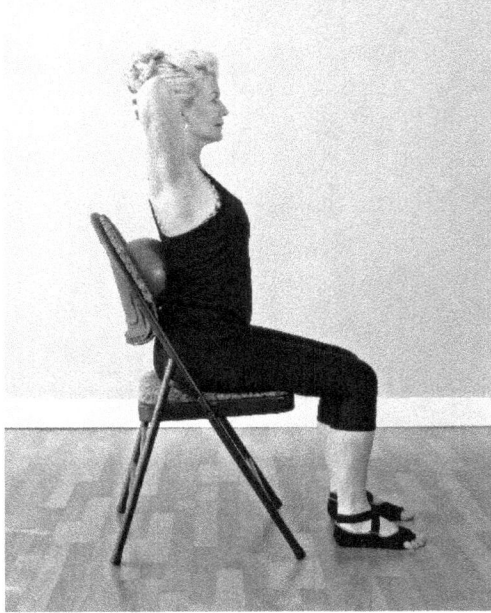

Slide your shoulder blades down your back. Bring your elbows into your peripheral vision

Exhale; pull belly towards the spine

Inhale; lift upper body (from sternum) over the ball to stretch the front of the spine.

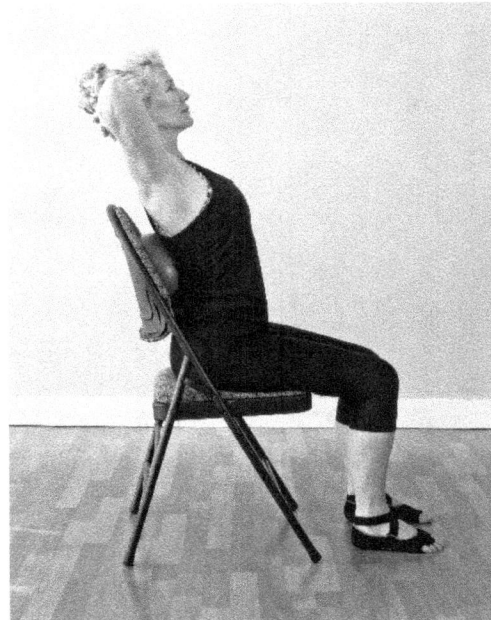

Exhale; pull belly to the spine and curl your spine forward, pressing your ribcage down.

Repeat 8-10x

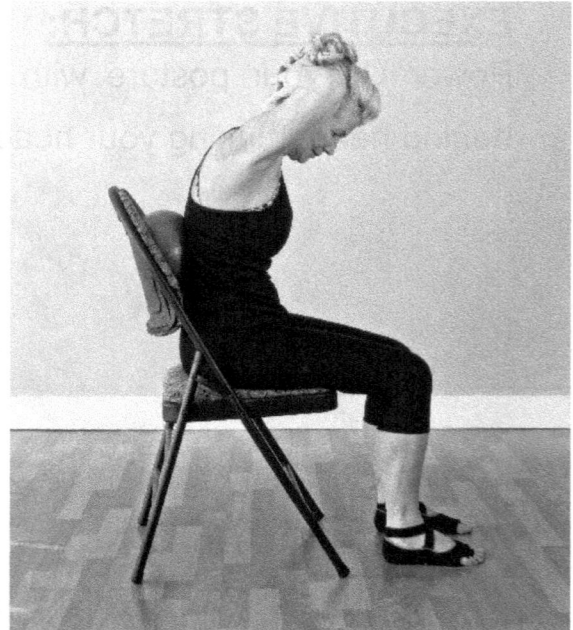

BENEFITS: Awareness of flexibility and mobility in spine, core strengthening.

PRECAUTIONS: Don't push on your head when curling spine forward.

HAMSTRING RELEASE

Power Up posture against the chair and then hinge forward from your hips. Rest your right foot on the ball.

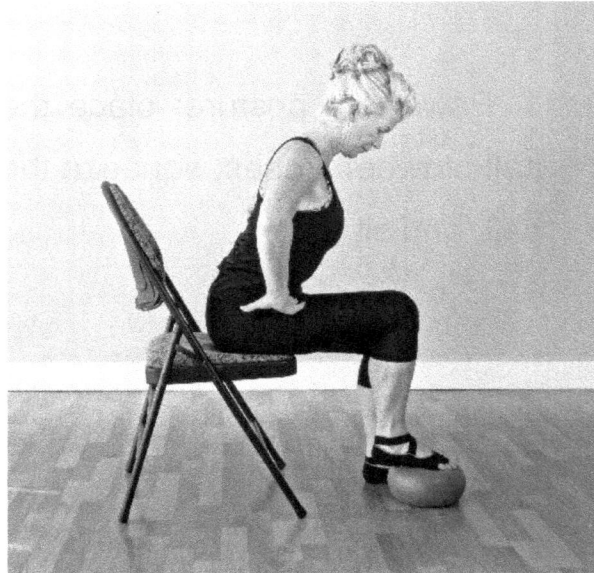

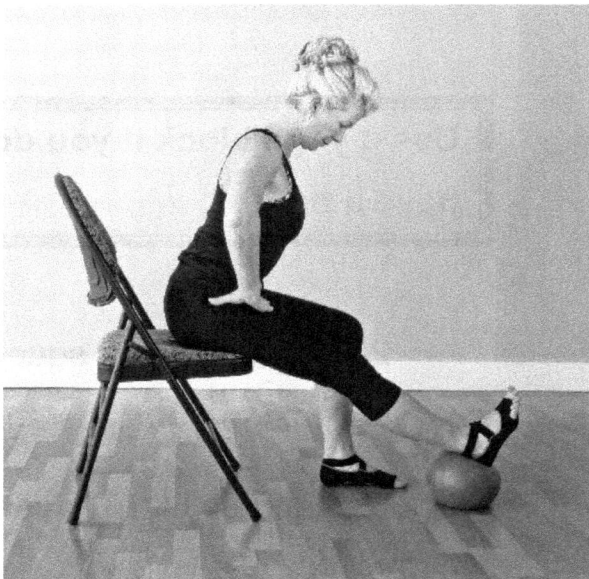

Exhale; pull belly towards the spine and roll out the ball, straightening your leg, pressing your heel into the ball and flexing your foot (toes towards the nose).

Inhale; roll the ball back in.

Repeat 5-8x increasing the stretch in the back of your leg each time. Repeat with left leg.

BENEFITS: To lengthen the backs of your legs; increase balance awareness and promote posture.

CHAIR (Utkatasana) POSE

1. Power Up posture; place the ball between knees, squeeze the ball, and sit tall.

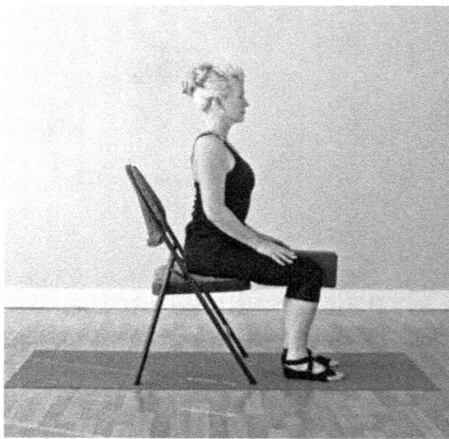

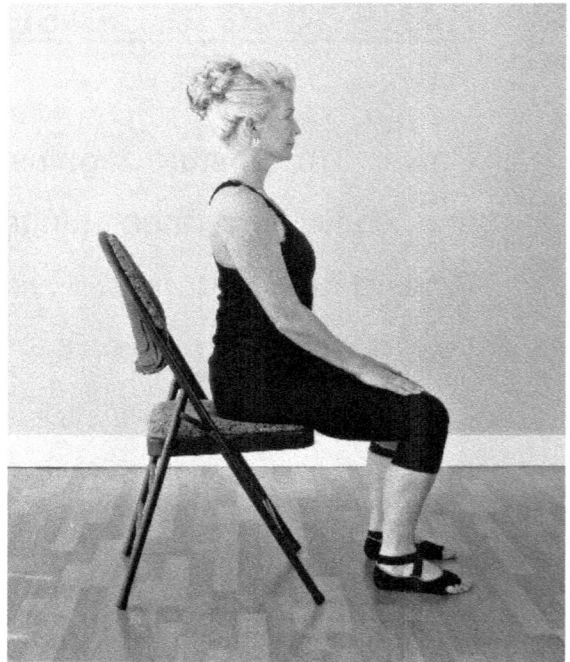

Use a yoga block if you don't have a ball.

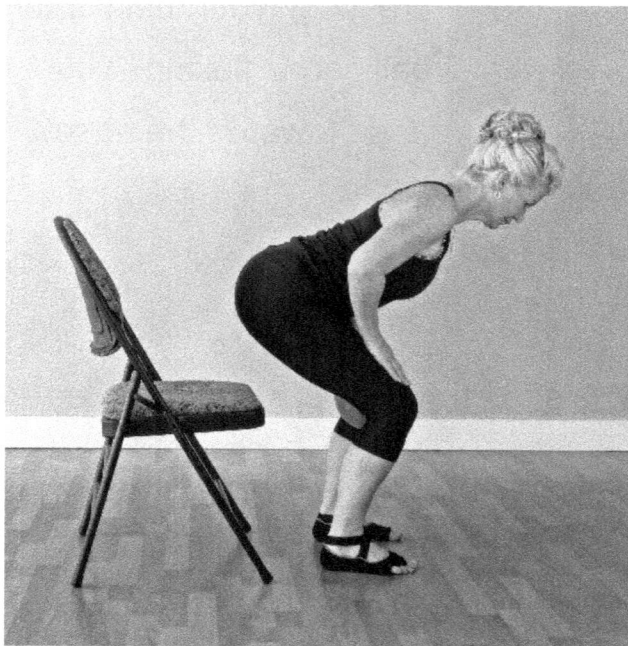

2. Exhale, belly in, squeeze ball, hinge from hips and

3. Stand up into **Tadasana**

Sit down and repeat steps 1-3 five times more

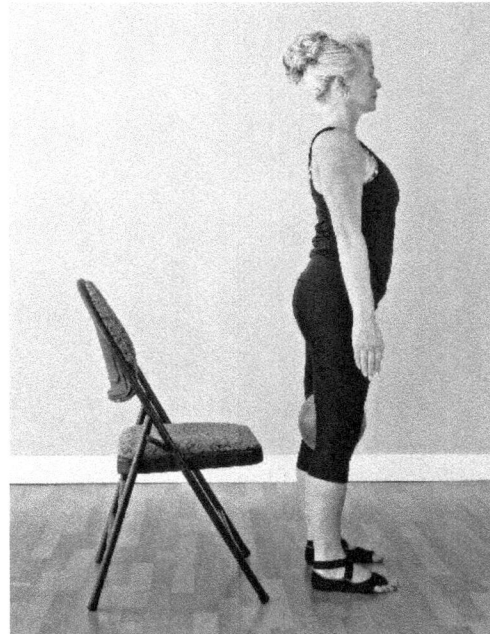

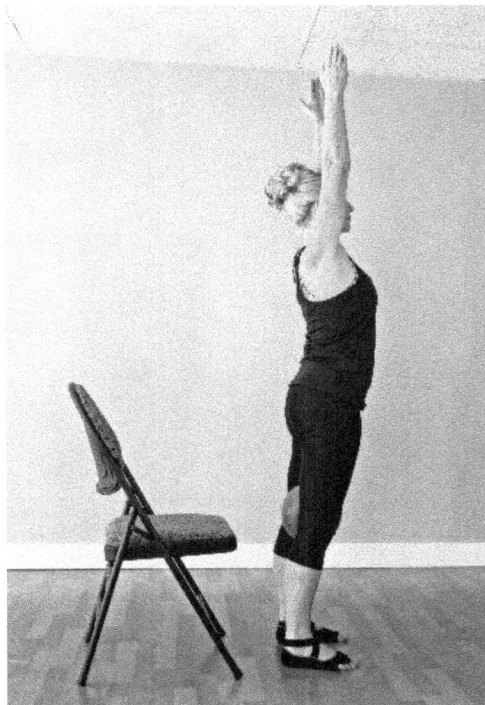

Inhale; Exhale and reach arms up and open (only as high as you can keep your shoulders down).

Hold for 3-5 breaths, squeezing ball.

Return to Sitting.   Relax for 2-3 breaths.

Come to standing behind the chair.

BENEFITS: Strengthens ankles, thighs, calves, core and spine;

PRECAUTIONS: Low blood pressure/High blood pressure - don't take arms overhead

CHAPTER 7

STANDING FLOW

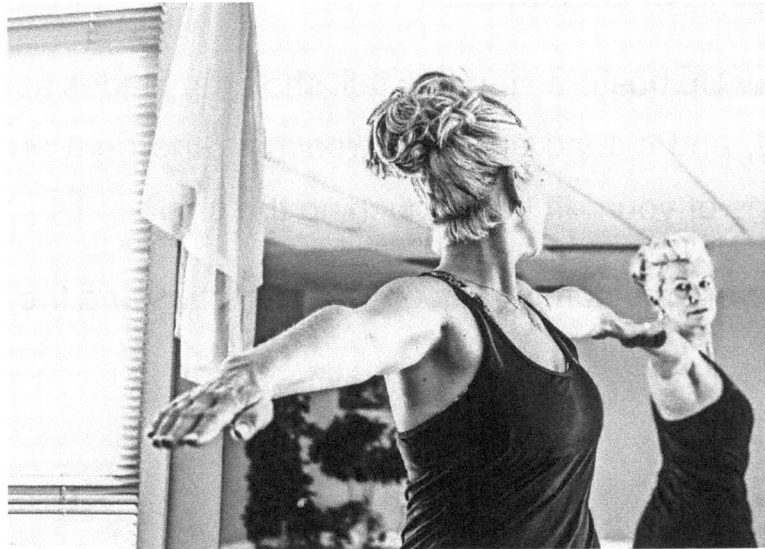

A Vinyasa is a transition of yoga poses put together to form a flow, coordinating the breath with the movement. Performing a Vinyasa helps to remind you that your muscles are fluid and that you need to keep moving. By setting your body up in a safe, balanced position, you are setting yourself up for success each time. ☺

If you have a yoga mat, place it on the floor and put your chair on top at one end facing the short end of the mat.

WARRIOR II (Virabhadrasana II)

1. Place left foot between the back-chair legs and step back with the right foot, aligning your left heel with the arch of the right foot. Press through the outside of your right foot (but keep the weight evenly through the foot) to promote the arch in the foot. Tighten your legs from the feet up.

2. Power Up posture standing tall, shoulder blades down and pulled forward, and extend arms out, reaching the right arm behind and fingertips of your left hand touching the chair.

Feel the energy coming out of your fingertips and the crown of your head.

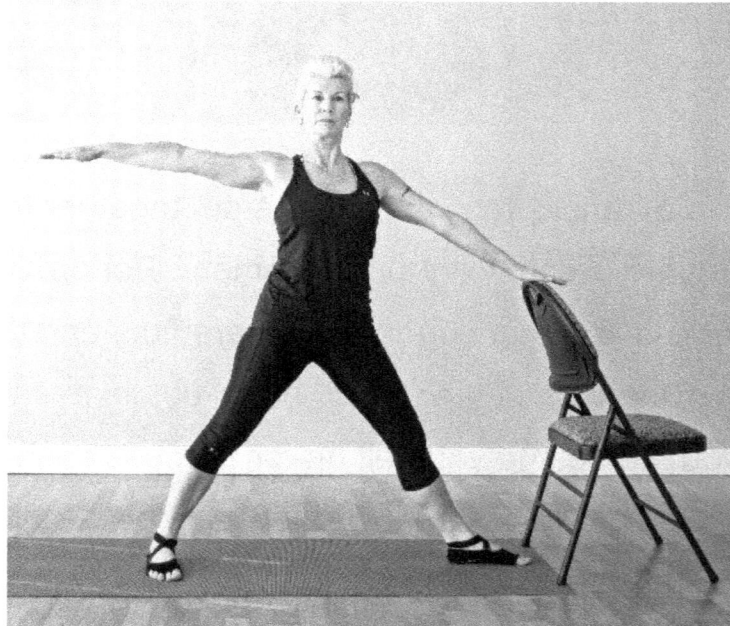

Inhale; pull the belly towards the spine

3. Exhale; bend left knee over top of the ankle, making sure the knee is pointing forward, and the weight is pressing through the heel to the ball of your left foot. Hold for 3-5 breaths.

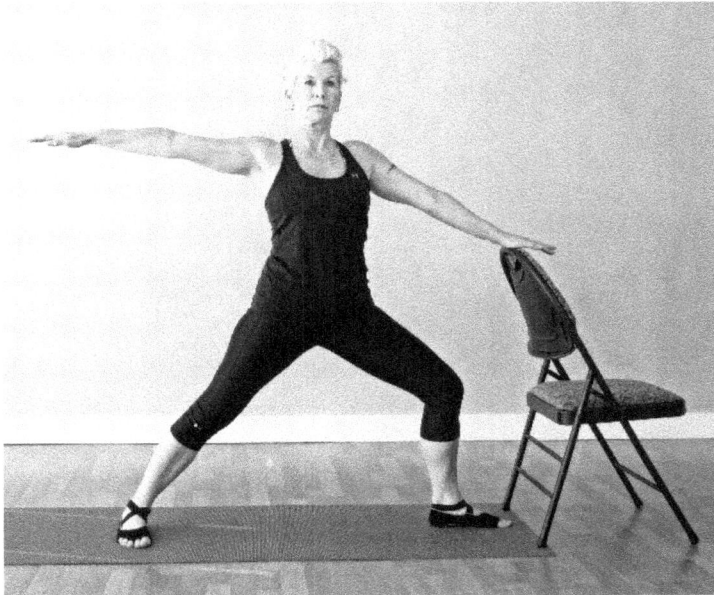

SIDE ANGLE (Utthita Parsvakonasana) POSE

1. Exhale; bend your left elbow down towards your left knee. Keep your left knee in line with the toes.

2. Inhale, move your right arm up towards the ceiling; relax your bottom shoulder.

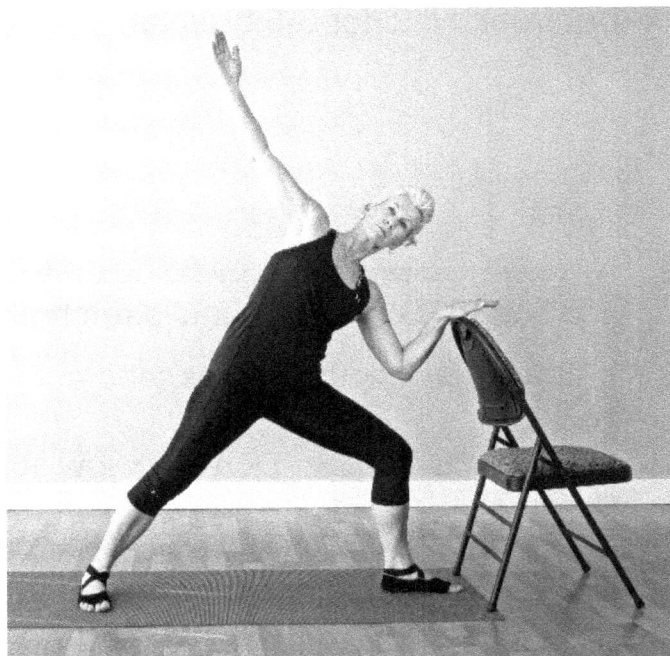

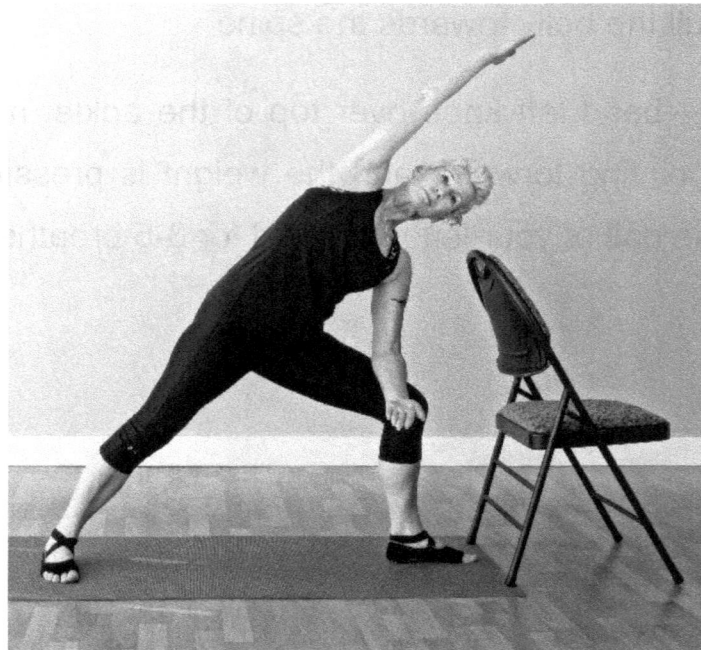

3. Exhale; move your right arm over your ear, creating a straight line from your right heel to fingertips. If you can, bring your left elbow to your knee and move your hand from the chair and hold out front. Hold for 3-5 breaths.

BENEFITS: Opens and stretches side of body from feet to fingers, strengthens legs, and energizes the body

PRECAUTIONS: Don't go low if there is any pain in your hips/knees. Drop arm if you experience pain in the neck or shoulders. High blood pressure - don't take arms overhead

Place your left hand on the chair and then windmill your right hand down to the chair as well, turning your chest to face the chair. Stabilize your shoulders, pull belly in towards the spine, and push yourself up to standing into

MOUNTAIN (Tadasana) POSE

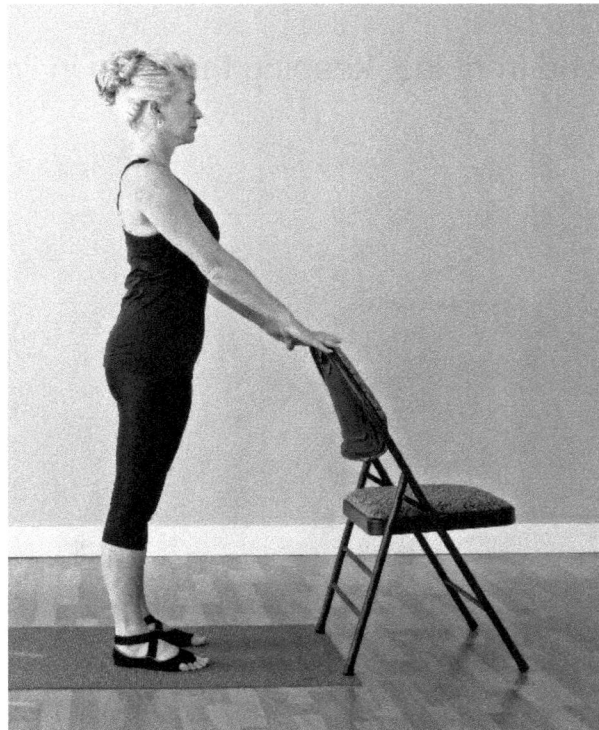

Take a few moments to find your balance and your breath. Tighten the legs from the feet up, regaining your posture.

WARRIOR I (Virabhadrasana I)

Step back again with the right foot, aligning heels, and right foot turned 45-60 degrees.

1. Inhale, magnetize legs, belly towards spine and shoulder blades down and forward.

2. Exhale; bend front leg, keeping the knee in line with toes.

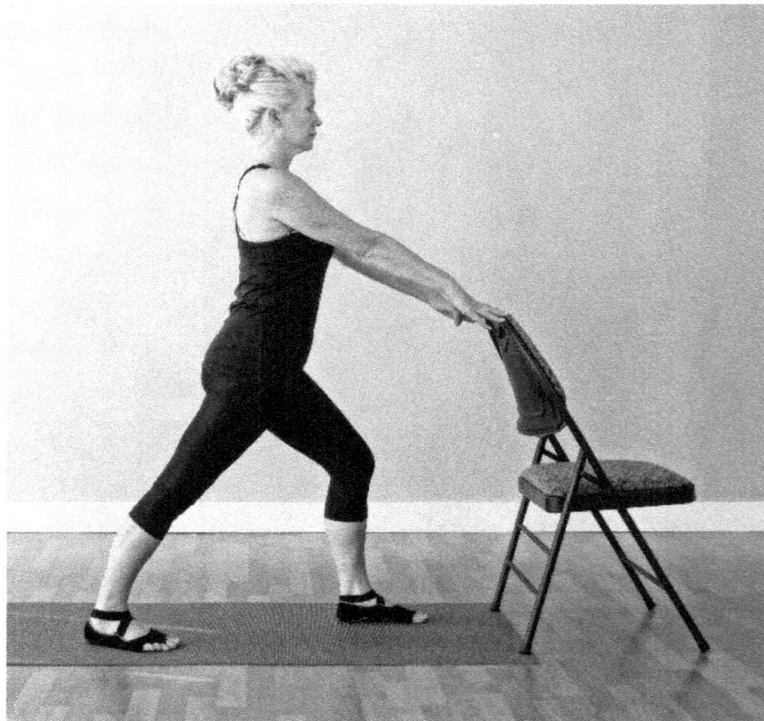

3. Inhale

4. Exhale; take one or both hands off the chair and reach towards the ceiling. Hold for 3-5 breaths.

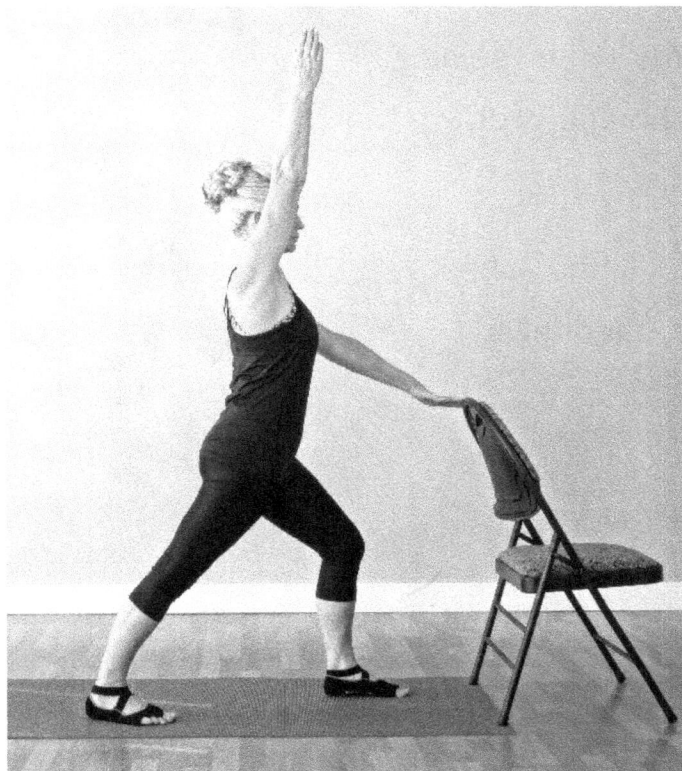

Bring hands back to the chair and step your right foot in, tapping the toes to the floor.

Steady your gaze and take 2-3 breaths.

.

BENEFITS: Strengthens legs and spine, lengthens hip of back leg, opens chest

PRECAUTIONS: Don't raise arms if you have any shoulder problems or high blood pressure.

WARRIOR III (Virabhadrasana III)

1. Tighten up legs, pull the belly towards your spine and slide shoulders down and forward.

2. Inhale; lift the chest, making you stand taller.

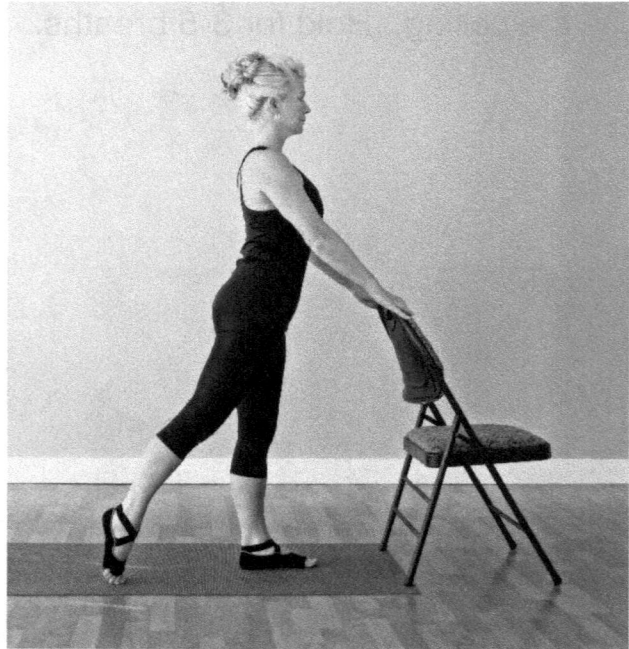

3. Exhale; tip from your hips, creating a straight line from the crown of your hand to the tips of your right toes. Move your hands to the seat of the chair. Hold for 3-5 breaths.

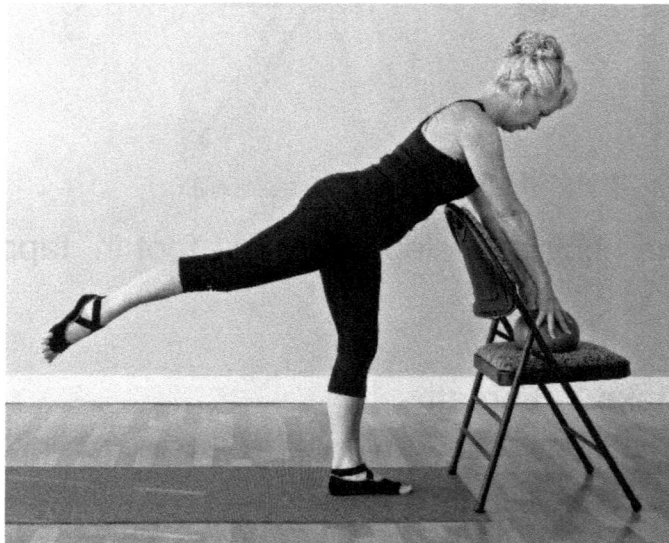

BENEFITS: Strengthens legs and spine, promotes posture, opens hip of back leg.

PRECAUTIONS: Keep hands on back of chair if your balance is compromised

CHALLENGE: PLACE BALL UNDER HANDS

When you're ready, pull belly towards the spine, and come back to **Mountain (Tadasana) Pose**. Steady your gaze and hold for a few moments, connecting with your breath.

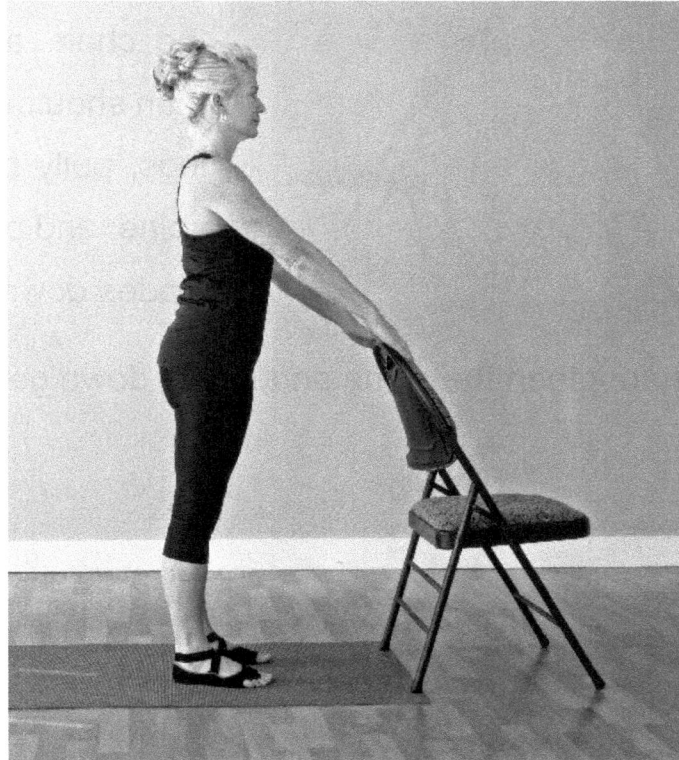

REPEAT THE STANDING FLOW SERIES WITH THE

RIGHT FOOT FORWARD:

Warrior II ~ Side Angle Pose ~ Tadasana
Warrior I ~ Warrior III ~ Tadasana

DOWNWARD-FACING DOG (Adho Mukha Svanasana)

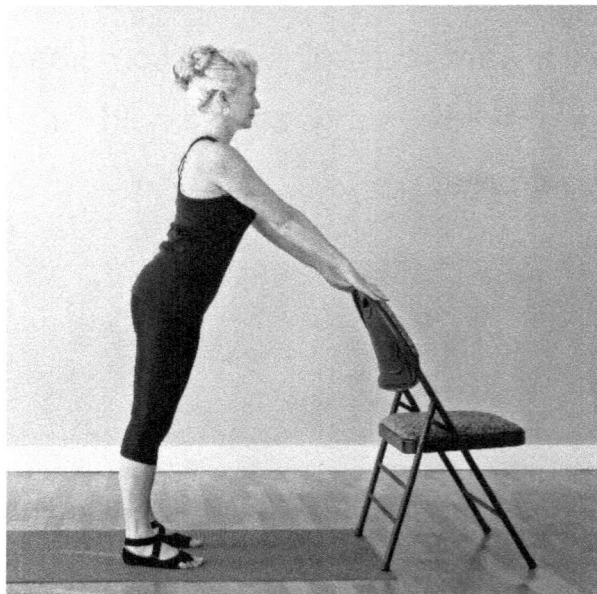

Step back 2-3 feet away from the chair, feet hip-distance apart, hands on the back of the chair, and a little wider than shoulders. Tighten your legs, pully belly towards the spine, and pull your shoulder blades down and forward.

1. Inhale; lengthen the spine and, press down gently through your hands.

2. Exhale; push your hips back, pressing your heels into the floor. Slide your shoulder blades down your back, creating space between your ears and arms; keep your spine long. (Try to touch the wall behind you with your hips). Hold for 5-8 breaths, breathing into sides of ribs.

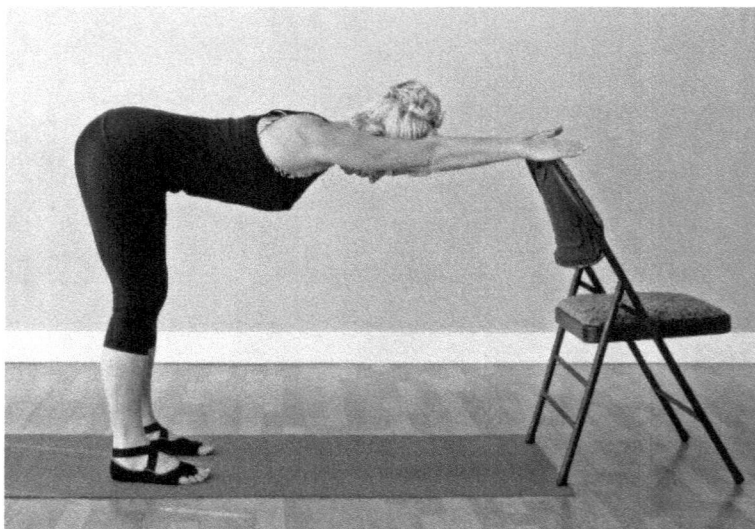

PRECAUTIONS: High blood pressure? keep your head in alignment with your arms or higher

CHAPTER 8

BALANCE FLOW

CALF RAISES

Stand with feet hip-width apart. Tighten legs, pull belly towards the spine, Power Up posture, slide shoulder blades down, and latch forward. Stand tall.

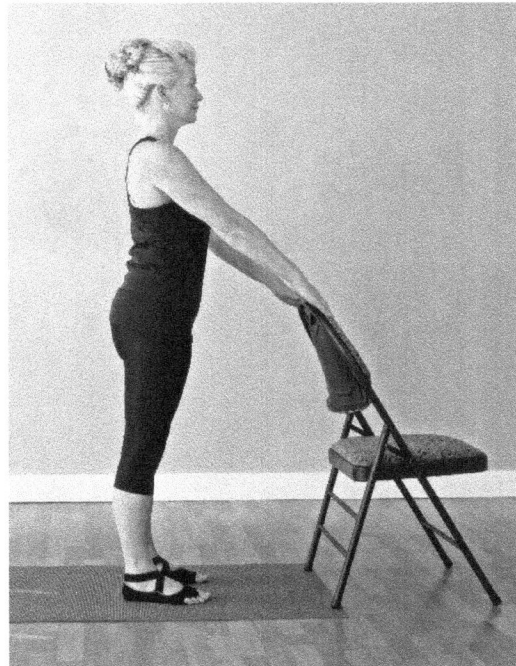

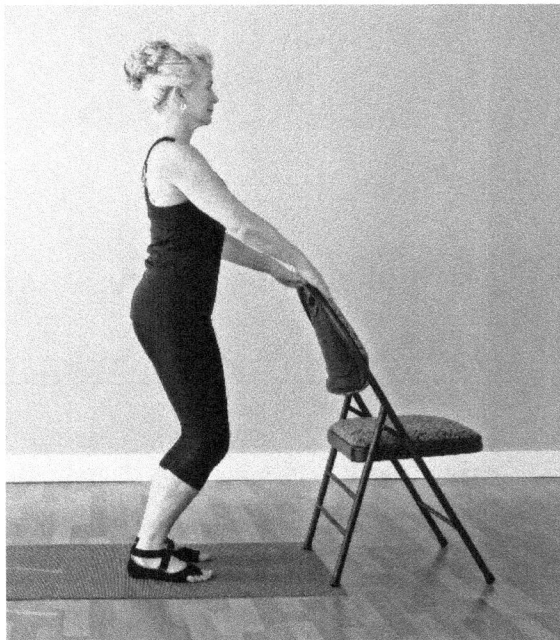

1. Inhale; bend knees

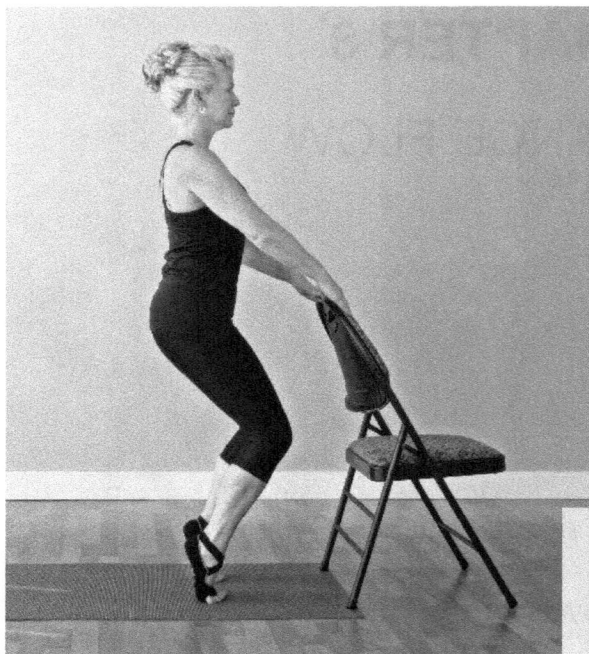

2.   Exhale, and lift heels, coming onto the balls of your feet

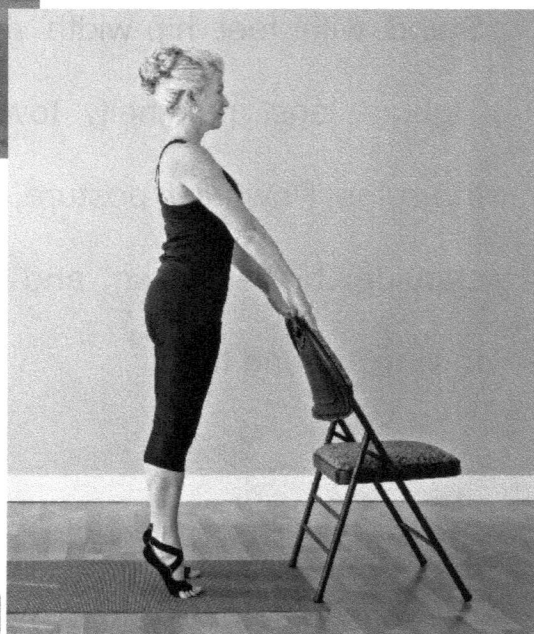

3. Inhale and straighten legs

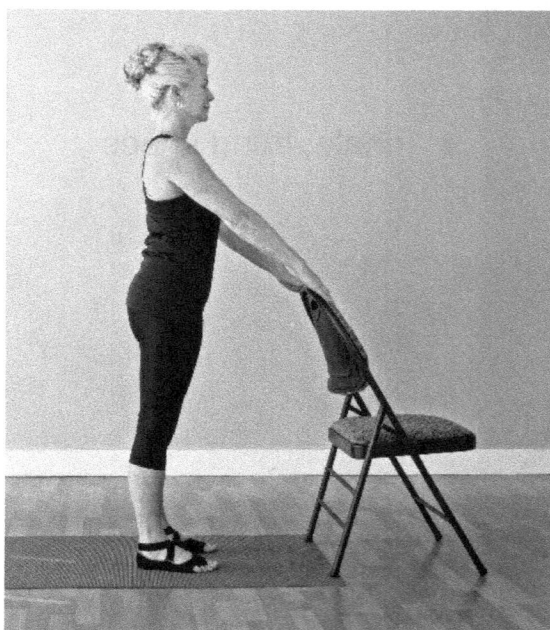

4. Exhale and slowly return to **Mountain (Tadasana) Pose**.

Repeat steps 1-4 three times more

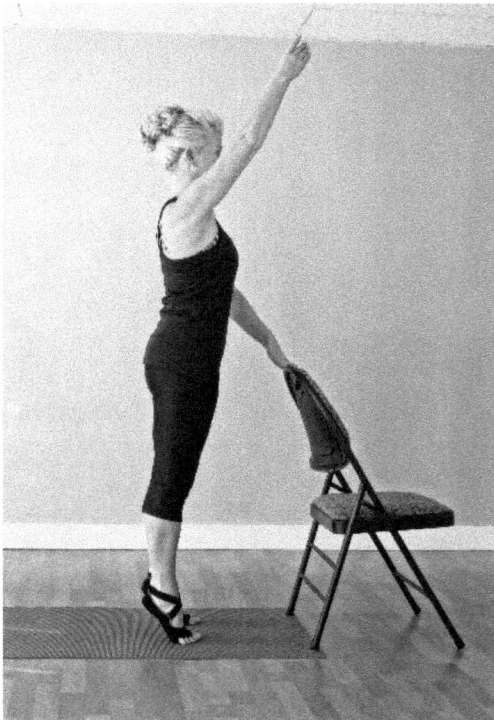

5. On the 4th time, stay on the balls of the feet and lift one hand away from the chair. Keep a steady gaze and stand as tall as you can.

Breathe into the ribs and hold the pose for 3-5 breaths. Bring your heels back to the floor.

Repeat step 5...this time lifting the other hand away. Hold for 3-5 breaths.

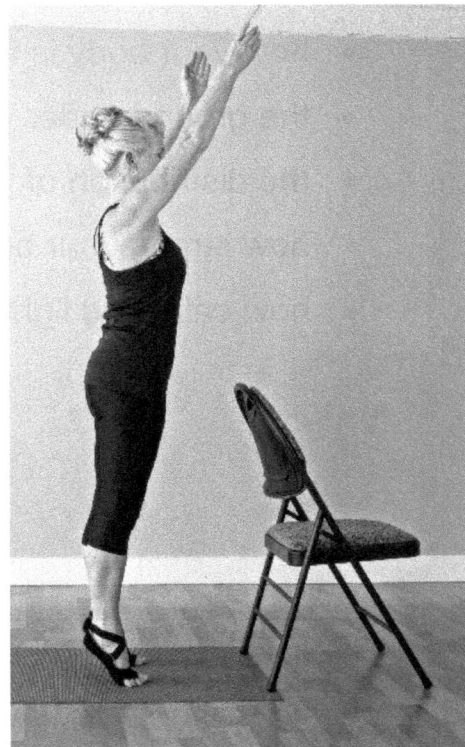

Bring heels to floor and arms to the chair coming into **Mountain (Tadasana) Pose**. Connect with the breath for a few moments, steadying your gaze.

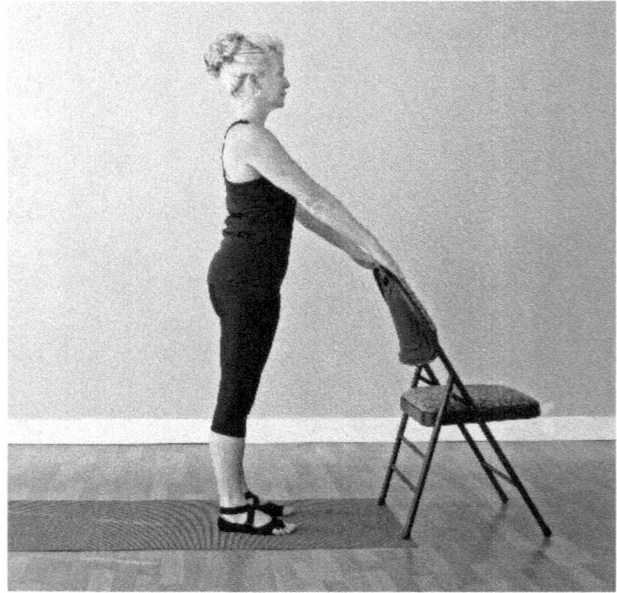

NOTICE:

- how your body is feeling
- the ground under your feet
- the distribution of your weight on your feet
- how strong your body is feeling
- how calm and light your breath is.

BENEFITS: Strengthens feet, ankles, calves. Broadens the chest. Promotes posture, balance, and core.

PRECAUTIONS: Keep hands on back of chair if balance is compromised

TREE (Vrksasana) POSE

Stand in **Mountain (Tadasana) Pose** to the right of your chair, about 6" away and touch fingertips to the backrest of the chair. Tighten up your legs, pull your belly towards your spine, and slide your shoulder blades down and forward.

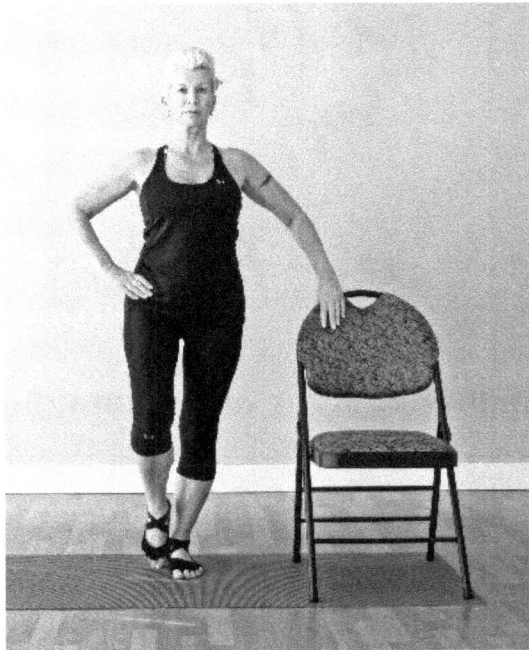

1. Glue your left foot to the floor, shift your weight slightly onto it, and bend your right knee, bringing your right foot up the outside of your calf, just below the knee.

2. Place the sole of your foot against the side of the leg, bringing your heel slightly forward, toes pointing down. Keeping your hips facing forward, turn the knee out to the right, tightening buttocks.

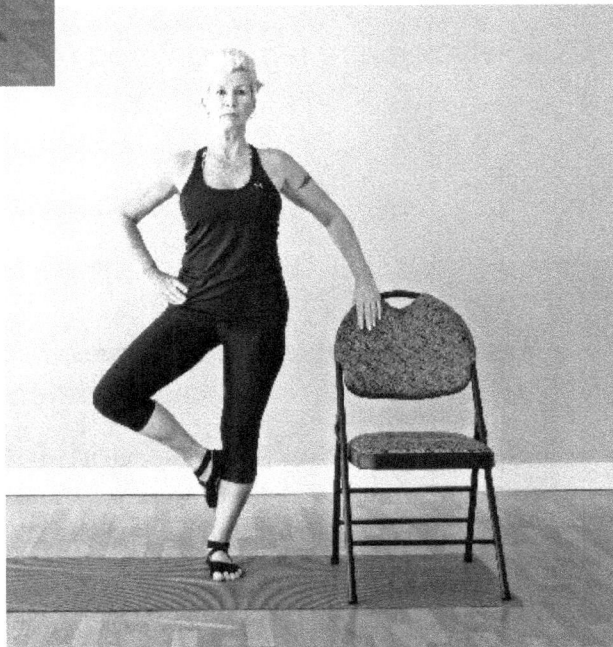

3. Keep standing tall pushing through the left foot and keeping belly to spine, bring right hand in front of the heart.

Steady your gaze and hold for   5-8 breaths.

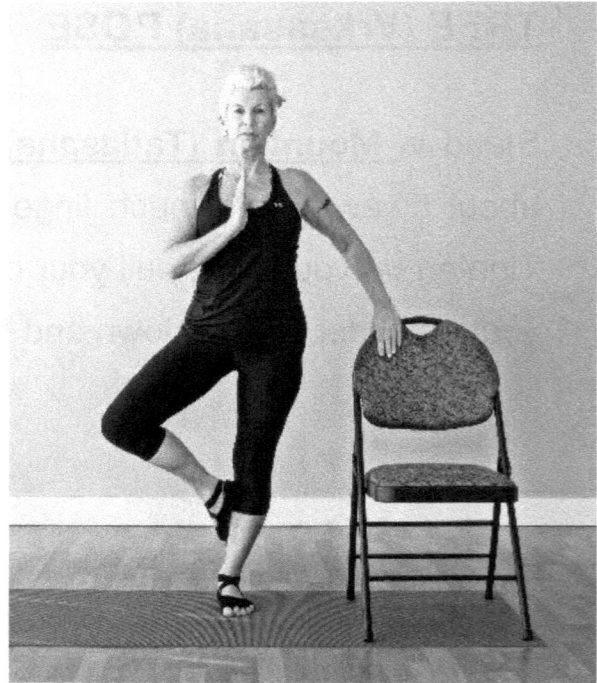

CHALLENGE: Raise hand higher until the arm is straight.

Slowly release leg and when ready, repeat on the other side.

BENEFITS: Improves balance and posture, strengthens spine, thighs, ankles, and feet. Stretches groin and inner thighs, broadens chest and shoulders, and relieves sciatica

PRECAUTIONS: Low blood pressure. High blood pressure - don't raise arm overhead.

CHAPTER 9

TWISTS

When we walk, our body is meant to naturally twist at the waist, bringing the opposite hand and leg forward, and keeping the rotation in our trunk. This natural gait (walk) pattern helps us move with ease and grace.

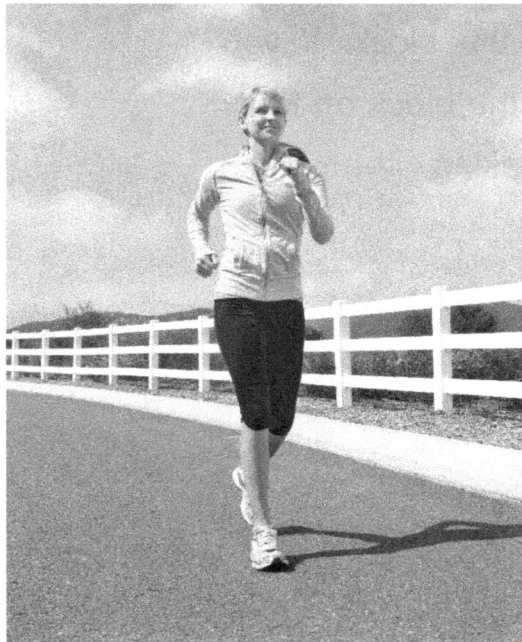

Restorative twists and poses can help prevent tightness and rigidity, two of the common symptoms of PD, by strengthening the core and increasing flexibility and mobility through the waist.

SEATED TWIST II

Take your feet quite wide and place a block in the center. Bring buttocks closer to the front of the chair and Power Up posture.

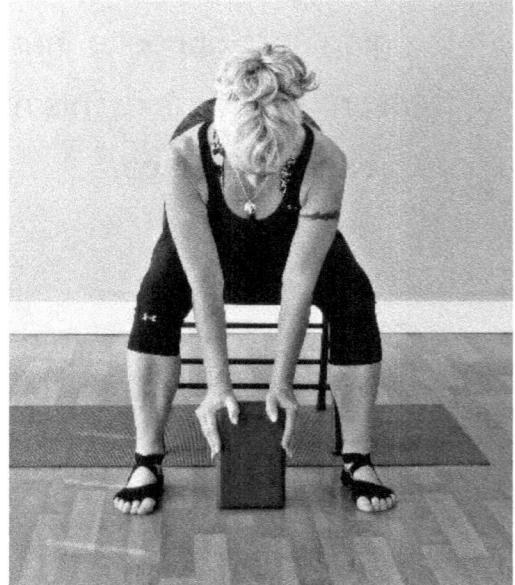

1. Pull belly towards the spine and hinge forward from hips, placing your hands on the block. If you can't reach, flip the block on to its short side, making the block higher.

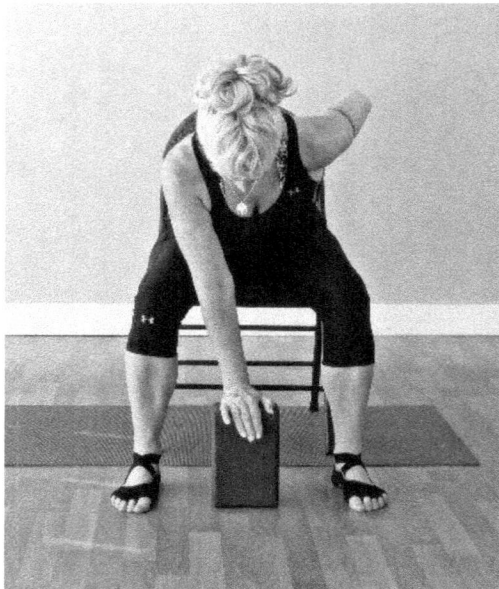

2. Roll your left shoulder back and place your left hand onto the small of your back.

3.   Exhale, pull belly to spine and begin to rotate at your waist, pointing left shoulder towards the ceiling.

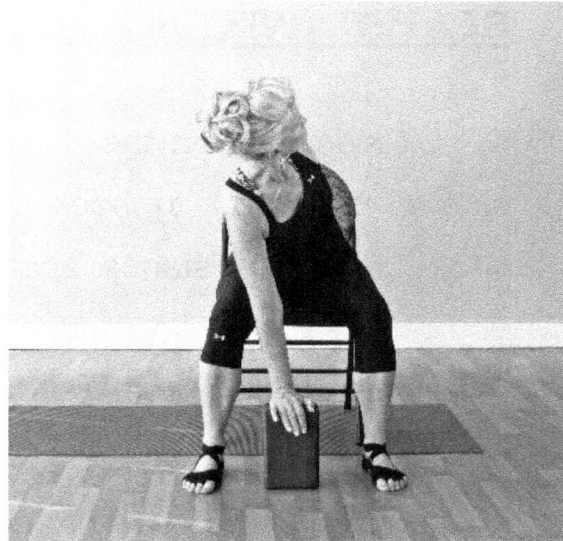

4. Continue reaching up with your hand. Hold for 3-5 breaths.

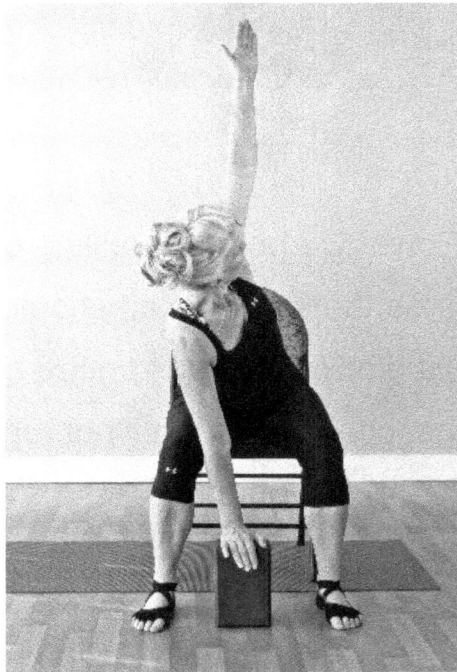

5. Inhale; bring your hand back to the block.

Pause; repeat with the right side

BENEFITS: Tones the abdominal organs, opens chest, increases mobility in waist, strengthens upper back

PRECAUTIONS: Low blood pressure, shoulder injury, tightness in back

SEATED TWIST III

1. Sit sideways on the chair (left side of the body to back of the chair), feet hip-distance apart. If you can't reach the floor, put a block under your feet. Place your hands on the back of the chair.

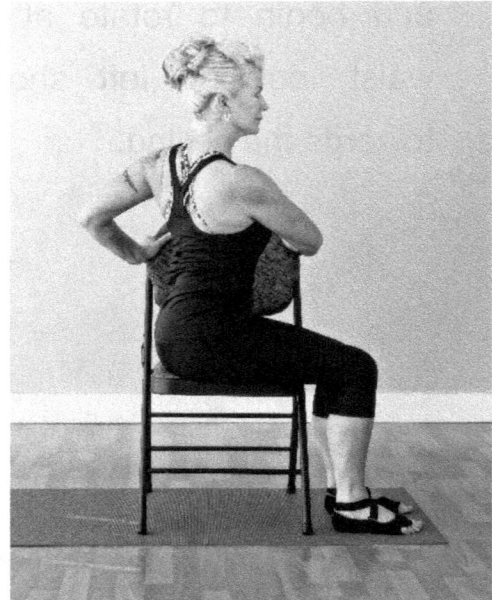

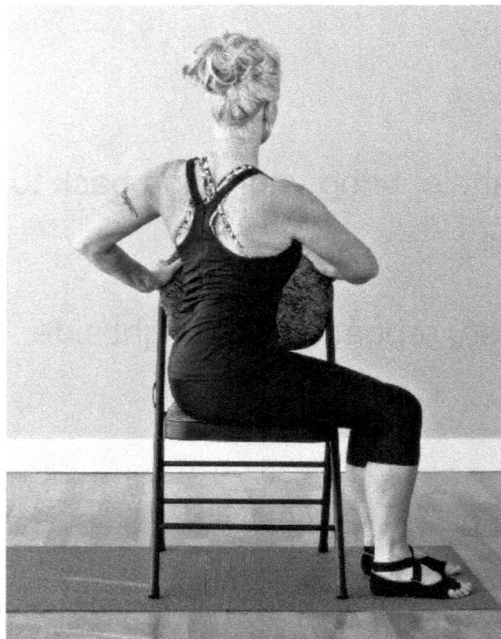

2. Power Up posture, pulling belly towards the spine, relax shoulders but lift elbows and pull on the back of the chair to widen your upper back and lift your chest.

3. Exhale; engage waist muscles and turn your belly to the back of the chair

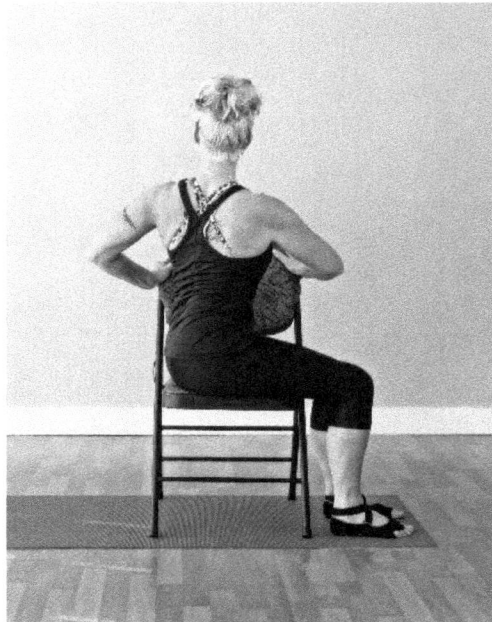

4. Inhale; pause. Sit taller and pull belly in towards the spine

5. Exhale; turn your ribcage to the back of the chair

6. Inhale; pause. Sit taller and pull belly in towards the spine

7. Exhale, turn your chest to the back of the chair

8. Inhale; pause. Sit taller and pull belly in towards the spine

9. Exhale, turn your head and look over your left shoulder.

To come out of the pose, release hands and gently untwist.

Take a resting breath before repeating on the other side.

BENEFITS: Eases spine and lower back, massages belly organs, improves digestion, strengthens abdominals

PRECAUTIONS: Only twist as far as it feels comfortable for you...

CHAPTER 10

THE FINALE

The last two poses, Cat Pose, and Cow Pose are a wonderful flow of movement that will bring the spine back to suppleness and ease spinal tension, bringing a wonderful finish to the practice. These poses are also known for calming the mind, opening the heart, and promote coordination of mind and body.

Sit towards the front of the chair. Power Up posture, place your hands above your knees with your elbows slightly bent and feet hip-distance apart.

Push through your feet to tighten legs, lengthen your spine, pull belly in towards your spine, and broaden chest; shoulder blades down and forward.

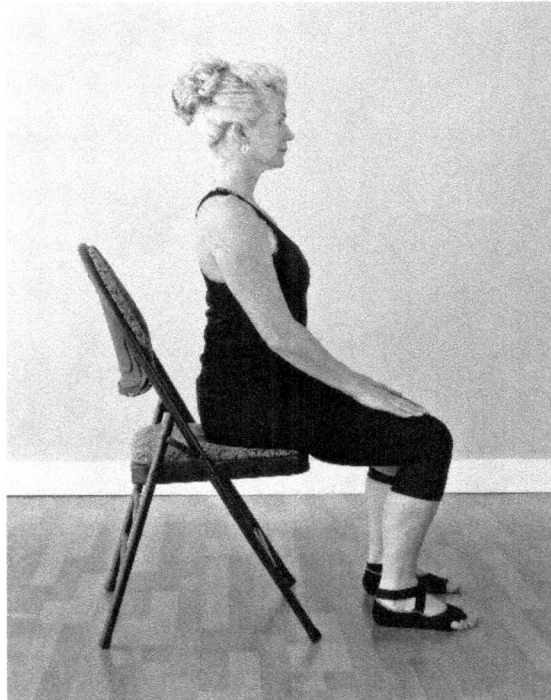

1. Inhale

CAT (Marjaryasana) POSE

2. Exhale; push away from your hands, rounding your spine one vertebra at a time, keeping the back of your neck long and in line with the torso

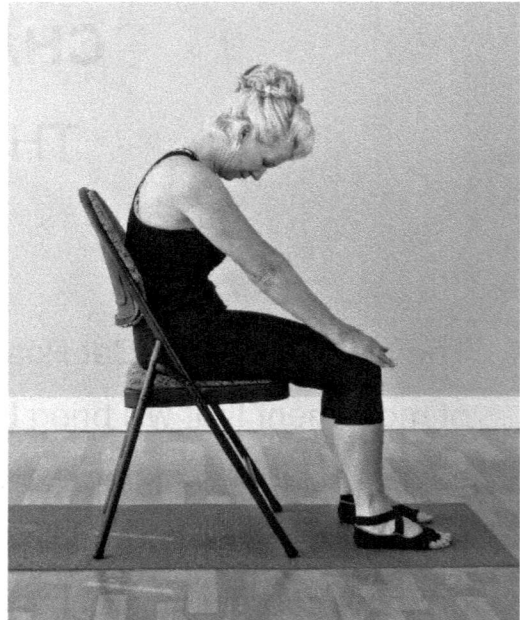

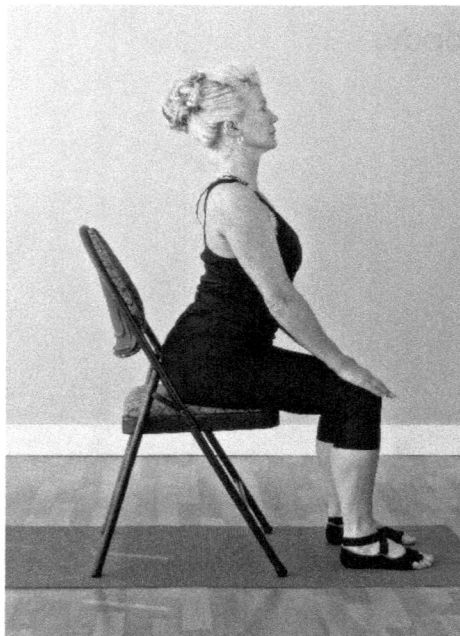

COW (Bitilasana) POSE

3. Inhale; lift your chest forward, creating an arch in your spine.

4. Exhale; come back into cat pose.

Repeat both poses 8-10x

BENEFITS: Stretches and strengthens the entire spine and provides a gentle massage to belly organs. Helps create emotional balance.

MODIFICATION: If knees fall out to sides, place ball between thighs to help keep legs tightened.

CHAPTER 11

COMING TO STILLNESS

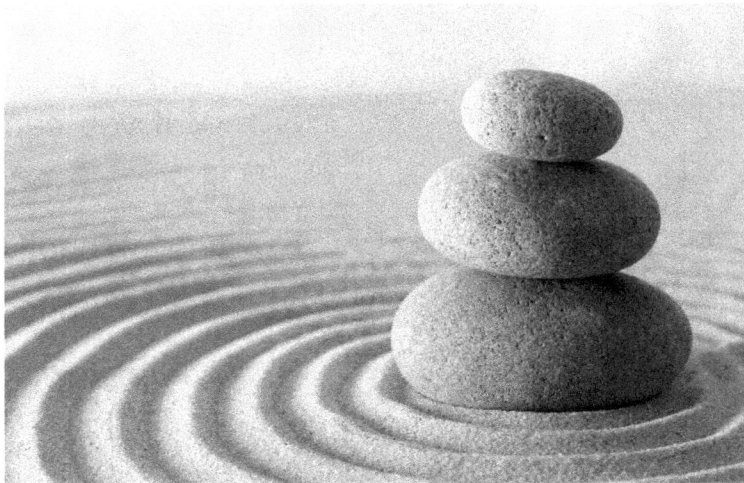

At the end of the yoga practice, around 7-10 minutes should be used for going into complete relaxation, allowing the body time to absorb the work of the practice, and to rejuvenate the body, mind, and spirit. Setting a timer for the allotted amount of time will allow you to go into relaxation without worrying about the time.

When we stop moving the body begins to chill so a sweater, socks and/or a blanket will keep you warm.

CORPSE (Savasana) POSE

There are many options on how to relax for your practice, and for PD, two positions of comfort are shown below. Choose the one that will allow you to stay comfortably in the position for about 7-10 minutes.

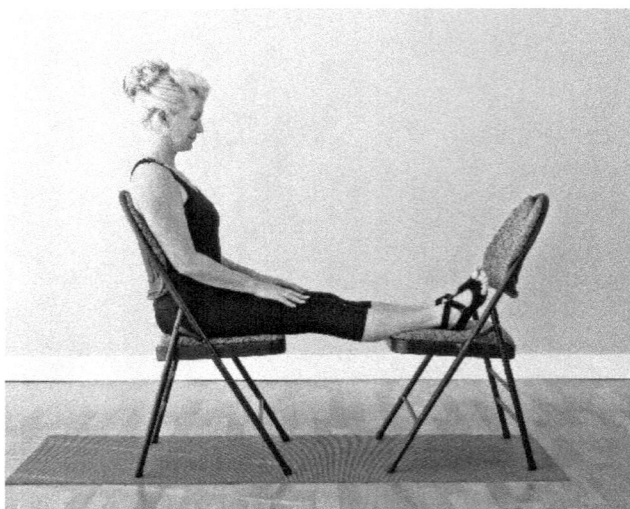

1. If you cannot get to the floor easily, placing your feet on another chair allows the body to relax completely.

2. If you can get down onto the floor, placing the feet and calves on the chair is a great way to relieve tired, aching legs. It helps open the front of the body and relieves any tension in the lower back.

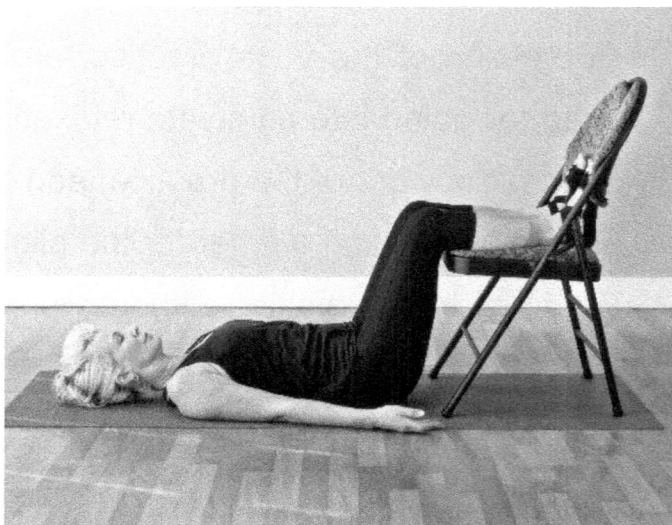

*Pillows or blocks may be used under the head if the neck buckles (the chin points up and back).

Whether lying on the floor or relaxing on two chairs, close your eyes and begin to breathe gently into the belly, noticing the belly rising and falling and allowing your body to relax.

The following meditation can be recited slowly into a recording device, (your phone or voice recorder) and then played each time you do the relaxation. An audio recording will allow you to focus on relaxing instead of trying to read each step.

The meditation has also been recorded by the author and is available as an audio download at www.rhonaparsons.com/balance-yoga-meditation

Listen to Rhona Parson's voice guide you through your relaxation so you can enjoy the benefits of letting go…

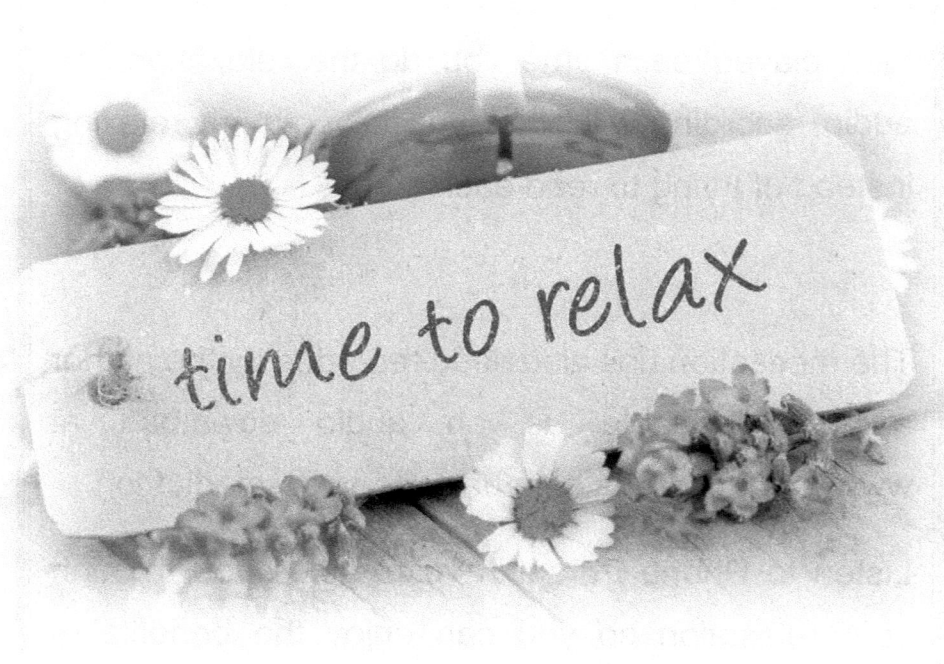

~RELAX, REST & RESTORE~

"Close your eyes and begin to breathe gently into the belly, noticing the belly rising as you breathe in and falling as you breathe out. As you breathe in, feel the cool air going in through your nostrils and as you breathe out, feel the warm air on your upper lip.

Breathe in… belly rises, breathe out… belly falls.

Allow your body to relax a little bit more with each breath.

Breath in…breath out…nothing more, nothing less. As the body gets heavier, the breath becomes lighter.

As you continue breathing and relaxing, scan your body with your mind's eye and notice if you're holding on to any tension somewhere. If you are, use the gentleness of your breath to release it.

Relax your legs, your belly; relax your shoulders, arms and hands…relax your face…your eyes falling deeper as your eyelids get heavier…jaw relaxed, so the mouth is slightly open; there is no expression on your face.

Sink deeper into the chair or the floor with each breath. Feel the heaviness of your bones sinking downward. Relax.

And now that you are in this peaceful, relaxed place, I want you to go to your favorite place; it could be your back garden, your favorite beach, it could be your favorite lake. It's where the sun is shining, the birds are singing in the trees, and wispy clouds are floating by. In this beautiful, peaceful place, it's just you, lying down or sitting completely relaxed.

Relax a little more and feel the warmth of the sun upon your skin. Breath in, breath out; nothing more, nothing less...Let go a little bit more.

Send your next breath to your heart and feel the warmth of your heart radiate throughout your body; from the crown of your head to the tips of your fingers and toes...

Sink a little deeper...any thoughts that enter your mind, acknowledge them, and then attach them to one of those wispy clouds and let them float away...Relax...sink a little deeper...feel the heaviness of your bones and notice the lightness of your breath...

Relax and let go ~~~~~~~~~~~~~~~~~~~~~~~~~~~~

Belly gently rises as you breathe in and falls as you breathe out.

Body relaxing…

Feeling the warmth of the sun upon your skin and hearing the birds singing in the trees.

It's such a peaceful, happy place where you are…

It's just you and your breath…………peacefulness; nothing more, nothing less.

Belly rises, belly falls, and your body sinks deeper.

It is now time to carry on with our day, so on your next exhalation, bring your awareness back to the room and your body. You're your mind's eye, see the room you're in, see the walls, see the floor, see your body lying or sitting.

Connecting with your body, gently move your fingers and toes, arms and legs, and when you're ready, go into your favorite stretch, stretching your entire body...

Take your time and when you are ready, come to a sitting position and let your head gently fall towards your chest, stretching out your spine and your neck. Bring your head back to center and slowly move your head side to side. Come back to center and gently turning your head side to side.

Open your eyes and take time here for you to gather your thoughts and bring back awareness.

Notice how you feel — coming back to the breath, noticing the belly rising with the breath and falling when you breathe out.

Together, we bring our hands touching in front of our hearts. Take a big breath in and as you:

Exhale...reach your arms forward, stretching your upper back. Feel the roundness in your upper back.

As you breathe in, open your arms out to the side to stretch your chest...reaching your arms back.

As you breathe out, reach your arms to the sky creating space between ribs and hips...coming up into our Power Up posture and then slowly, bring hands back down to your heart.

Breathe in and breathe out once again, reaching your arms forward to stretch your upper back.

Inhale...open your arms out to the side to stretch your chest...reach back behind you.

Exhale…reach your arms to the sky creating space between your ribs and your hips...and slowly bring your hands back to your heart center.

As always, we close our practice with Namaste

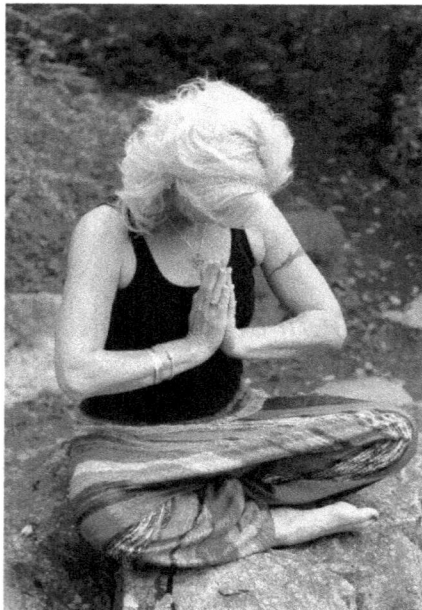

"the light in me honors the light that is in you also...."

I am blessed. Thank you

Rhona ♥

CHAPTER 12

STRETCHING WITH THE YOGA STRAP
AND MODIFICATIONS

The Yoga strap is a great tool in yoga as it helps prevent muscle or joint strain and enhances the stretch that you are doing.

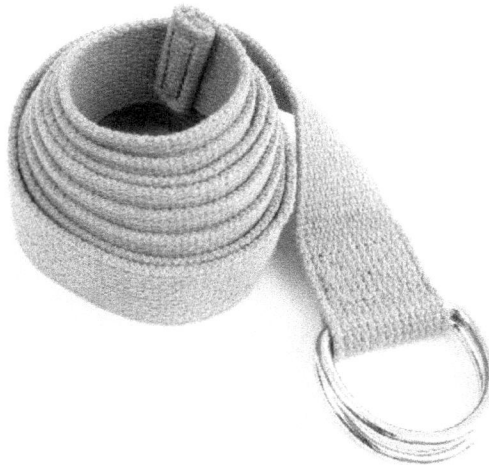

In Yoga Balance, the strap allows you to ease into a deeper stretch that you normally would not be able to do because of tightness or rigidity in your muscles. The strap creates "longer arms" and aids you in being able to hold a pose longer than normal.

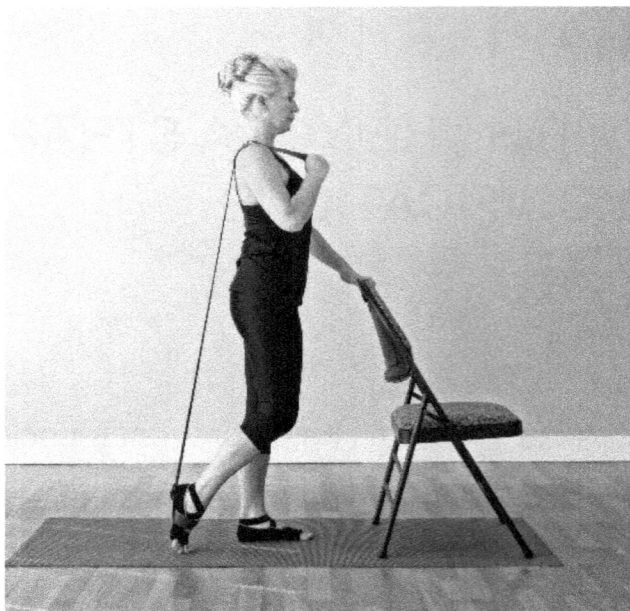

FRONT OF THIGHS

Set up as shown with the yoga strap looped around the right foot (buckle at the back of the foot) and the end of the strap draped over your right shoulder.

Hold on to the chair with your left hand for balance.

(This can also be done by sitting on the chair and allowing the leg to hang off at the side)

Exhale; slowly pull on strap, bending the knee and lifting the foot. You should feel a stretch down the front of your thigh.

Inhale; lower.

Repeat lifting and lowering four times more. Lift and hold, focusing on balancing and pushing through standing leg.

Hold for 3-5 breaths.

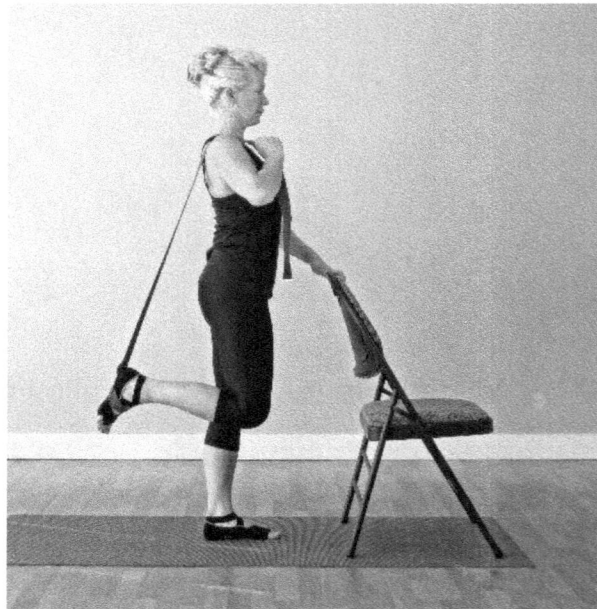

MODIFICATIONS

KNEELING ON CHAIR

Set up as shown with left knee on the front of the chair and holding on to the back of the chair with your left hand. Your right hand is on your hip to help with balance.

Exhale; gently push hips forward, tightening buttocks until you feel the stretch down the front of your left thigh. Hold for 3-5 breaths.

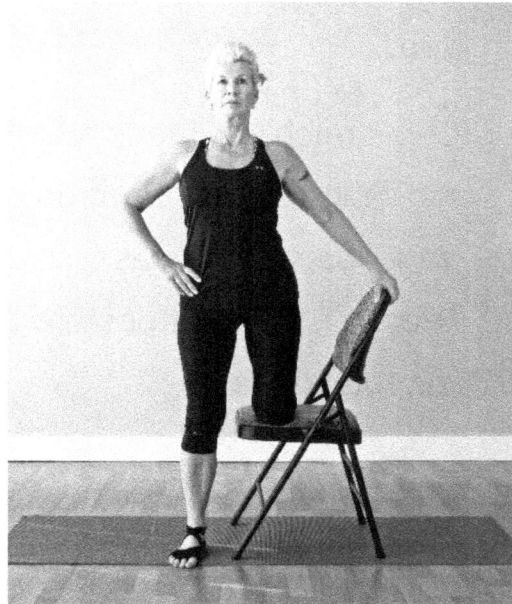

HIP AND CALF STRETCH

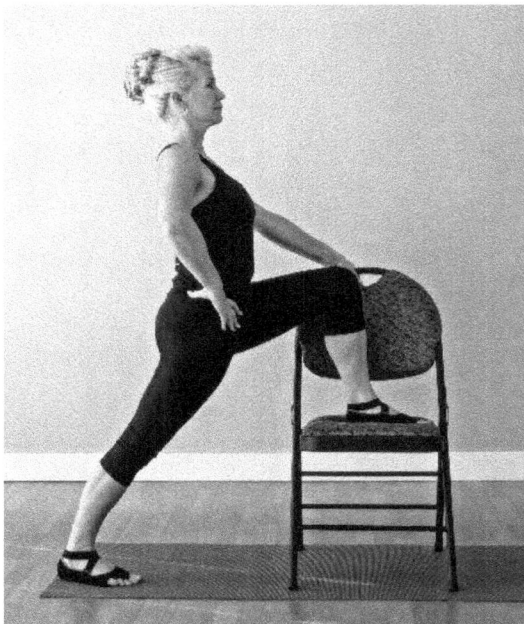

Set up as shown with left foot on the chair (knee over top of the ankle) and left hand holding on to the back of the chair. Point the right foot forward; heel in line with toes.

Exhale; push hips forward, and tighten buttocks. You should feel a stretch in your right calf area and at the front of your right hip. Hold for 3-5 breaths.

On your next breath:

Tighten the buttocks and lift your right arm, reaching back behind you.

The stretch will intensify in the right hip, and you will be strengthening your back muscles, creating a "Power Up" great posture position for your spine.

Hold for 3-5 breaths.

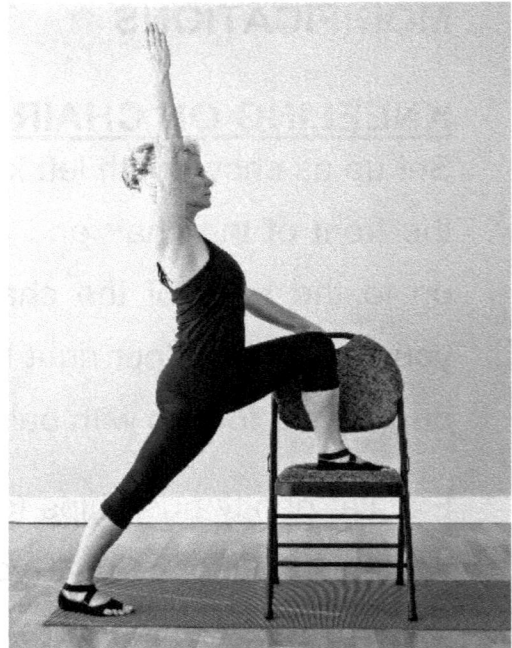

SIDE STRETCHES

Begin with Power Up posture, strap in both hands and hands wider than shoulders, held at chest height. Pull belly towards spine.

1. Inhale; slowly raise arms overhead

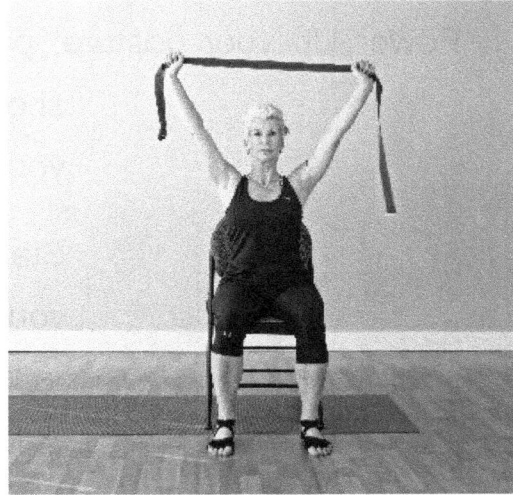

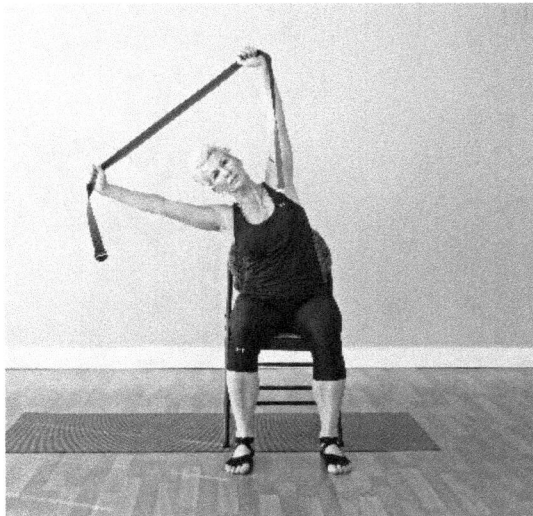

2. Exhale; keeping weight under both hips, pull on the strap with your right hand, tipping the upper body to the right

3. Inhale; back to the center

4. Exhale; tip to the left.

Repeat two more times each side.

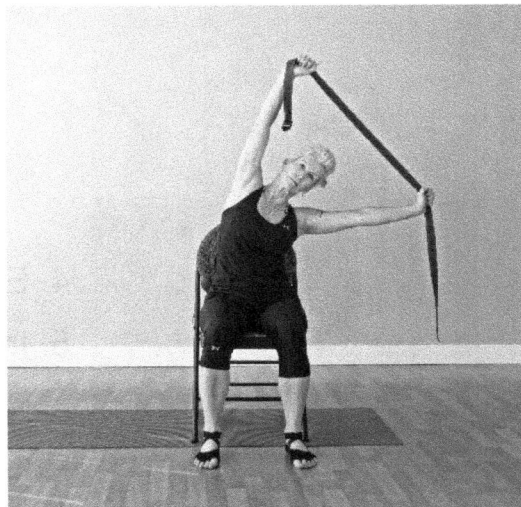

SHOULDER STABILIZATION

Make a loop with the strap, big enough to fit your hands and shoulder-width apart.

Power Up your posture, pull belly towards the spine, slide your shoulder blades down, and ground through your hips and feet.

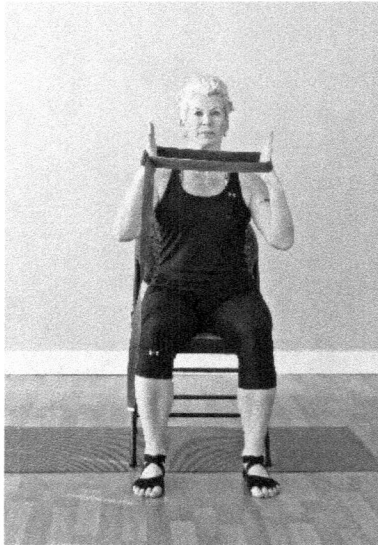

Stabilize your shoulder blades by pressing your hands into the strap:

1. Inhale

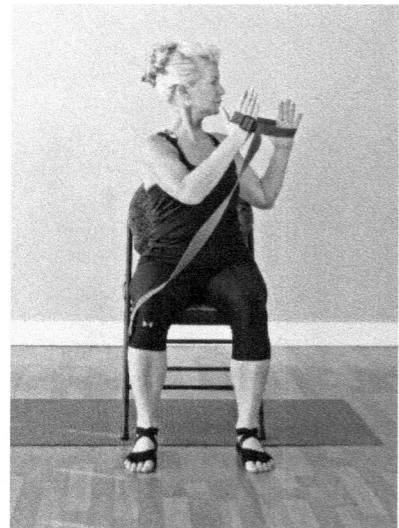

2. Exhale; twist upper body to the left
3. Inhale; come back to the center

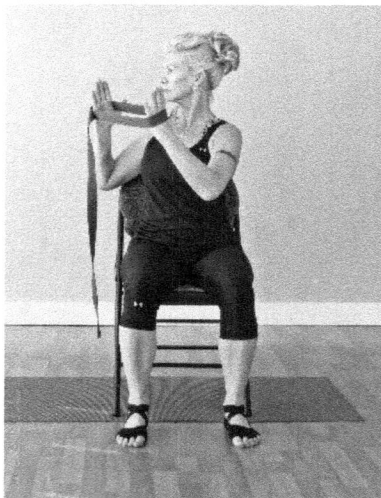

4. Exhale; twist to the right
5. Inhale; come back to the center.

Repeat two more times each side.

CHAPTER 13

STRETCHING ON THE FLOOR WITH THE YOGA STRAP

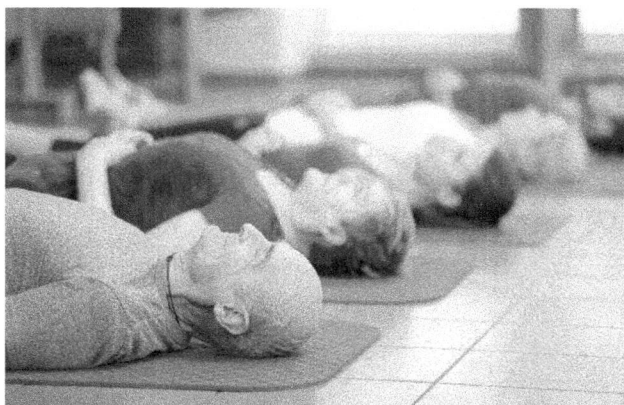

If you can get to the floor, these yoga stretches for your legs create alignment, length, and support using the yoga strap.

For some of us, our necks take a lot of strain and tension when we lie on the floor. If you are tight in your shoulders, have a rounded back or a short neck, chances are you have difficulty placing your head on the floor without your neck buckling (your head tilts backward, placing a lot of strain on the back of the neck). Place a pillow (or two) under your head to release the tension felt in the back of the neck.

In Balance Yoga, we apply a very simple exercise to create length in the back of the neck when lying on the floor. This lengthening, once mastered, along with allowing your eyes to follow the movement of your head, will help eliminate any tension in the neck.

NECK LENGTHENING

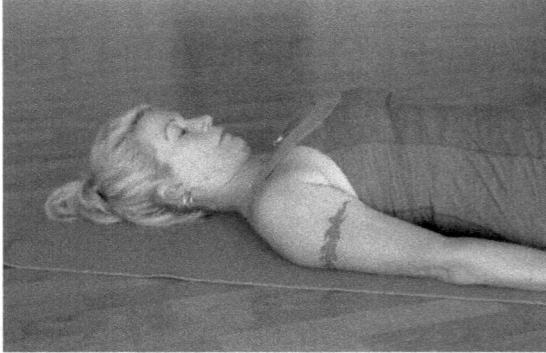

1. Inhale; keeping your head on the floor, lengthen the back of your neck (drop your chin down towards your throat). Make sure you don't jam your chin down.

2. Exhale; release back to the starting position.

Repeat 3-4 times, finishing with neck lengthened.

SHOULDER STABILIZATION

Stabilize your shoulder blades by this simple exercise. Make sure that the backs of your arms touch the floor throughout the movement.

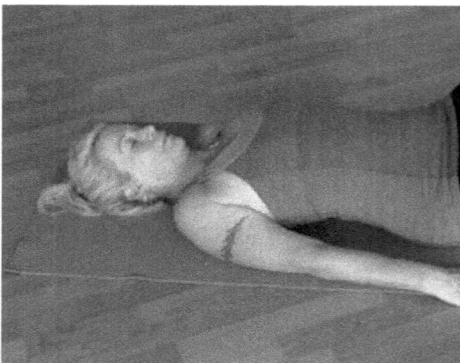

1. Inhale; elevate your shoulder blades

2. Exhale; gently press your hands into the floor and slide your shoulder blades into their place.

Repeat 3-4 times

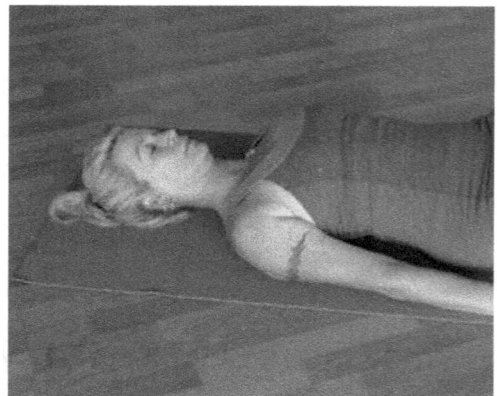

HAMSTRING STRETCH

Place yoga strap around your left foot and lie down on the floor; keep left leg down, and bend the right knee. Relax and lengthen your neck. Notice that your lower back is off the floor. (This is neutral).

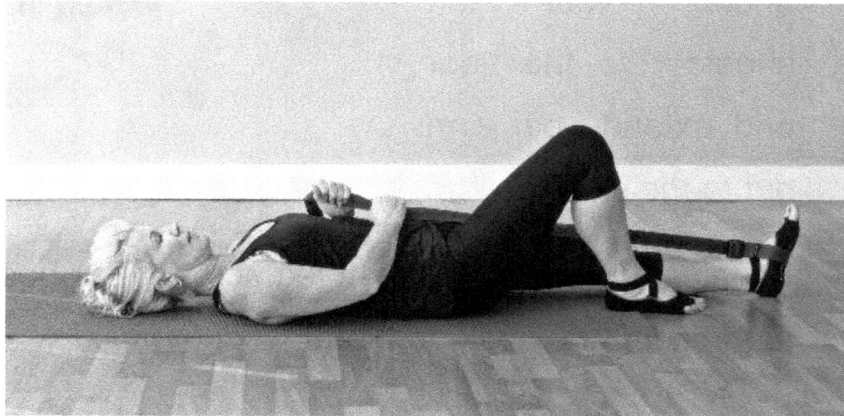

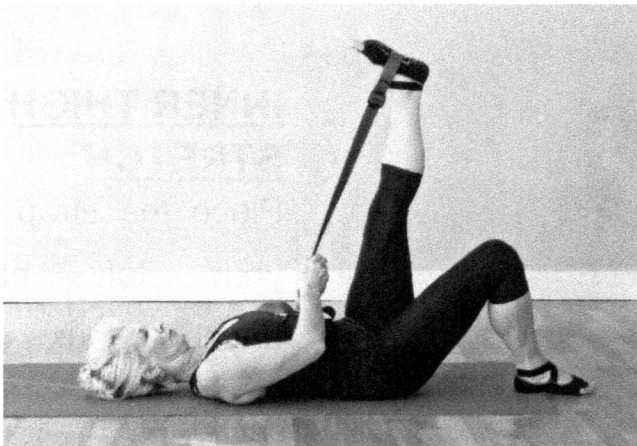

1. Keeping spine in neutral, slowly walk hands up the strap to lift the leg to hip height

2. Tighten buttocks and slowly lower leg down, sliding the strap through your hands) Repeat four more times.

3. Walk hands up the strap to lift the leg to hip height (keep neutral spine).

4. Leave the leg in the air and slide hands down straps, elbows to floor and hands resting on the body. Pull leg down into the hip socket and hold for five breaths.

SPINAL TWIST

Straighten your right leg. Place the strap into your right hand, anchor your left shoulder to the floor and extend your arm out to the side.

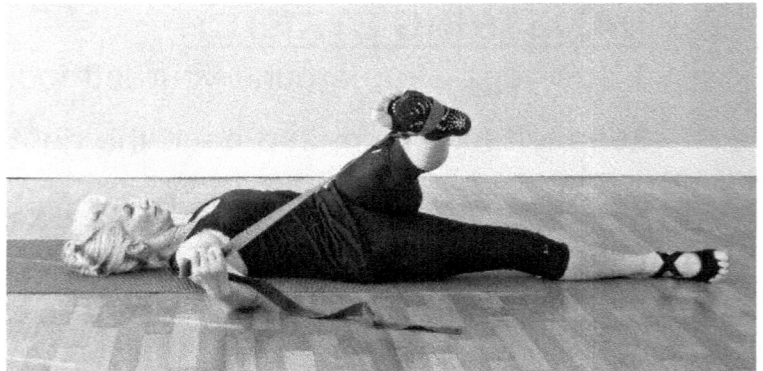

Exhale; Slowly pull your left leg across your body. Turn your head to the left (if no neck problems).

Hold for **five breaths**, allowing your leg to drop towards floor Exhale; Slowly roll onto your back, bringing the head back to the center.

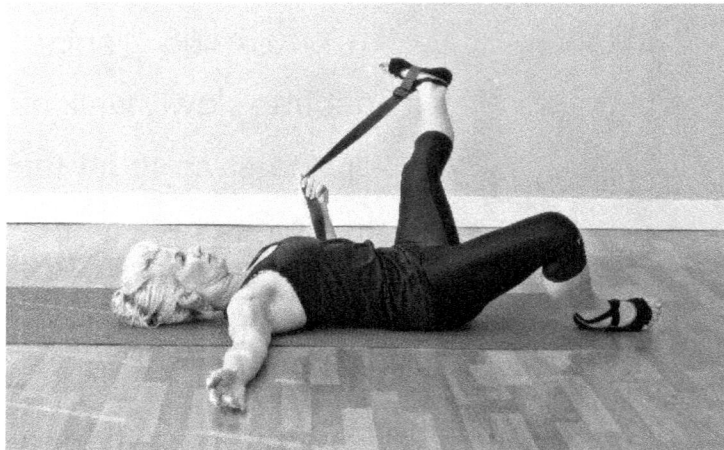

INNER THIGH STRETCH

Place the strap into your left hand, anchor your right shoulder to the floor and extend your arm out to the side. Anchor your left elbow to the floor and bend your right knee.

Exhale; Slowly let leg fall to the left; **at the same time,** let right knee fall out, keeping your pelvis even on the mat...hold for five breaths Exhale; Slowly roll onto your back.

HAPPY BABY POSE

Come up to sitting and make a bigger loop in the strap and place it around both feet. Slowly lower your body back onto the floor (head supported if needed), bend your knees into your chest, and straighten your legs.

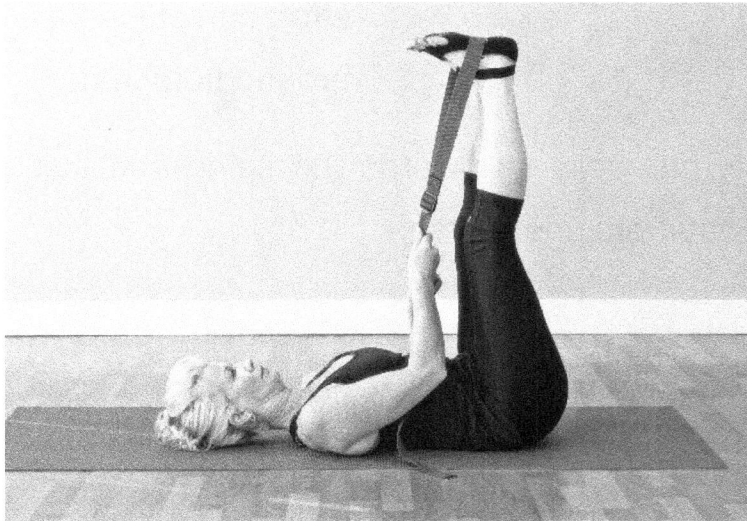

Push your feet into the strap to keep your tailbone on the floor and flex your feet (toes towards your nose).

Hold for five breaths.

Exhale; pull belly towards the spine (to anchor your back onto the floor) and slowly press your feet apart, **at the same time,** bending your knees in towards your chest. Hold for five breaths.

Slowly lower legs to the floor and rest for a few breaths.

REPEAT THE FLOOR STRETCHES WITH THE

RIGHT FOOT IN THE STRAP:

Hamstring Stretch ~ Spinal Twist ~ Inner Thigh Stretch

SEATED FORWARD FOLD

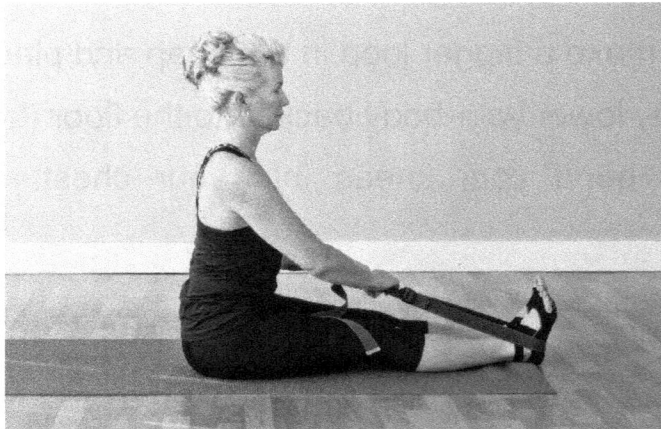

Sit on pillows or blocks if your legs are tight and your back rounds.

Undo the loop of the strap and place the strap around both feet.

Power Up posture, pull belly in towards the spine and pull your shoulders down away from your ears.

Inhale;

Exhale; hinging from hips, slowly walk your hands down the strap towards your feet.

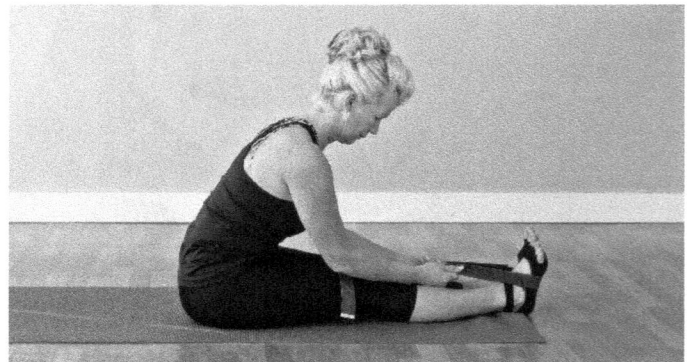

You will feel a stretch in the backs of your legs and your lower back.

Inhale; sit tall, walking your hands up the strap and stacking your spine one vertebra at a time

Repeat two more times and then stay forward and hold the stretch for five breaths.

CHAPTER 14

WHAT IS PARKINSON'S DISEASE?

Statistics show that PD is the second most common degenerative neurological disorder after Alzheimer's disease that affects approximately 1 in every 500 people in Canada. Today over 100,000 Canadians have PD, and over 6,000 new cases are diagnosed each year in Canada.

PD develops when there is a loss of nerve cells in the brain, which produce a chemical called dopamine. Dopamine is a neurotransmitter that controls the way messages travel from one nerve cell to another in the area of the brain, known as the substantia nigra, that controls muscle action. The cells that produce dopamine begin to die, reducing the amount of dopamine. When the loss of these cells reaches approximately 80%, the symptoms of PD appear. The disease progresses over time, as the dopamine levels in the brain gradually fall. The progression of the disease and accompanying symptoms vary with each person.

SUBSTANTIA NIGRA

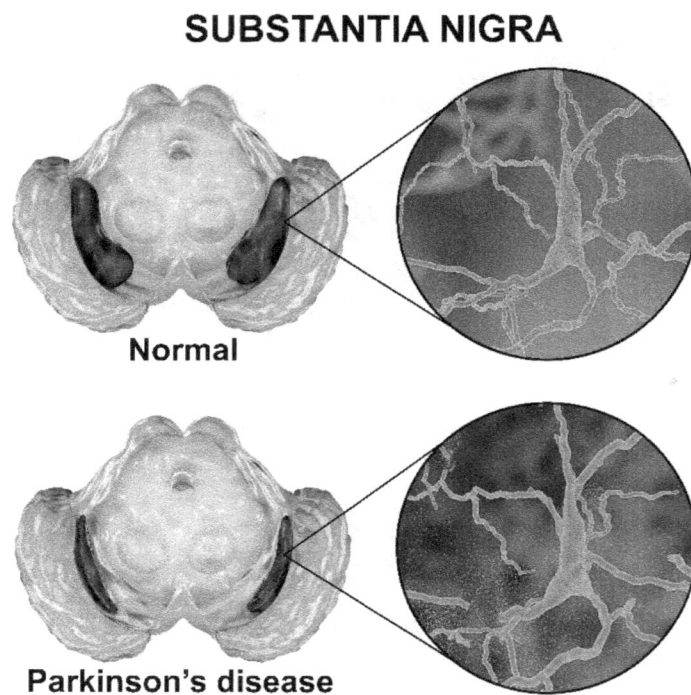

Normal

Parkinson's disease

Many of my clients say that when they look back at photos of themselves, they can see the "masked" face appearance that people with PD acquire over time.

THE MOST COMMON SYMPTOMS OF PD

Some of the chief motor symptoms that appear are:

- Slowness and stiffness
- Trouble with balance
- A tremor
- Rigidity of muscles

and non-motor symptoms include:

- Fatigue
- Sleep disorders
- Soft speech
- Depression
- Problems with handwriting
- Poor posture

"I often say now I don't have any choice
whether or not I have Parkinson's, but surrounding that
non-choice is a million other choices that I can make."

Michael J. Fox

CHAPTER 15

FREEZING WITH PD

Although the side effects of PD can differ significantly from person to person, many people with PD are particularly prone to feet problems because of difficulties they experience with walking (gait), posture and cramping in the feet.

Abnormal foot function can cause a lot of discomforts and, inevitably, can affect a person's mobility, putting them at more significant risk of falling. As the progression of PD becomes more apparent, a person's stride length begins to shorten, and the amount of time both feet remain in contact with the ground increases. This grounding can be one of the reasons for freezing.

Freezing is a temporary, involuntary inability to move. It can happen at any time, anywhere, and anyplace. It is where the weight of the body lands in the center of the feet and feels as though your feet are glued to the floor.

How can we help someone who freezes? Frank would always freeze in class, and when he did, he would ask me to place my leg in front of him at shin height so that he would need to "step over it." He asked me to place horizontal lines of duct tape on the floor going into the men's washroom at our gym because it was where Frank would freeze frequently. Every time he approached the doorway, he would "step" over the lines.

When George froze, I would give him a gentle nudge on the shoulder to "tip him sideways," releasing one foot from the floor by shifting his weight onto the other foot. After a few attempts, this would solve the problem for him.

Unfortunately, there is no known cause for Freezing.

When we walk, a 'normal' walking action is to touch the ground first with the heel and then finally push off with the toes. The gait is a 'heel-to-toe' gait.

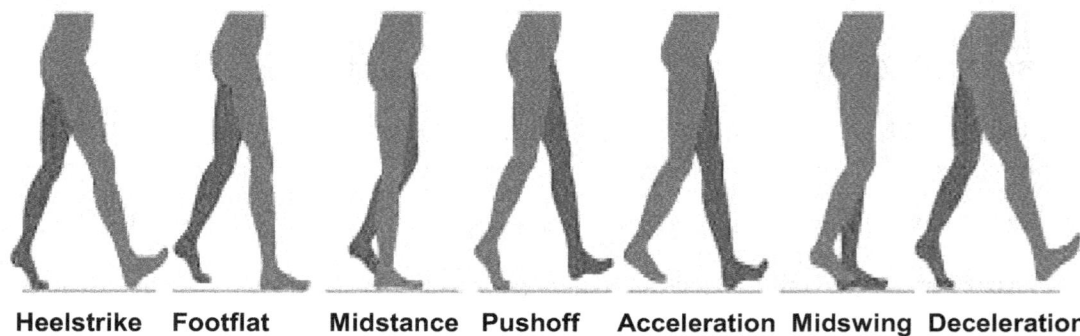

Heelstrike   Footflat   Midstance Pushoff   Acceleration Midswing Deceleration

When rigidity begins to happen within the ankle, the person with PD can often lose this normal heel-to-toe gait and starts to walk with a shuffling action. This more flat-footed type of pace can produce foot, leg, and even knee pain as well as significantly reducing the foot's ability to absorb the shock of ground contact adequately. In the long term, this type of uncompromising stance can severely impact on an individual's mobility. *www.parkinsons.org.uk*

CHAPTER 16

WORLD PARKINSON'S DISEASE DAY

"April 11th is World Parkinson's Disease Day. This annual awareness day raises awareness of PD and promotes a greater understanding of how this condition affects people.

April 11th was chosen because it is the birthday of Dr. James Parkinson, the English physician who described the disease in a paper entitled "An Essay on the Shaking Palsy," published in 1817.

The silver ribbon is a symbol for children with disabilities, PD, and mental illnesses.

The symbol of World Parkinson's Disease Day is a red tulip. This symbol dates to 1980 when J.W.S Van der Wereld, a Dutch horticulturist, developed a red and white tulip. Van der Wereld, who had PD, decided to name his newly cultivated flower the 'Dr. James Parkinson' tulip.

On April 11, 2005, the Red Tulip was launched as the worldwide symbol of PD at a conference in Luxembourg".

Eimear O'Brien, Brand Communications

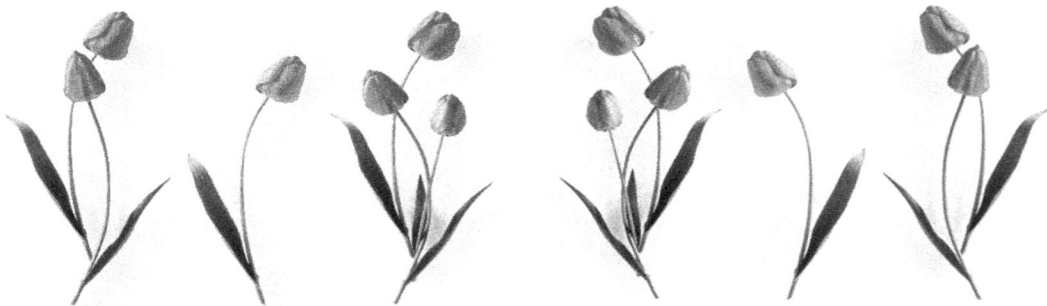

CHAPTER 17

ABOUT THE AUTHOR

"Inspiring Real Purpose and Real Change in the World"

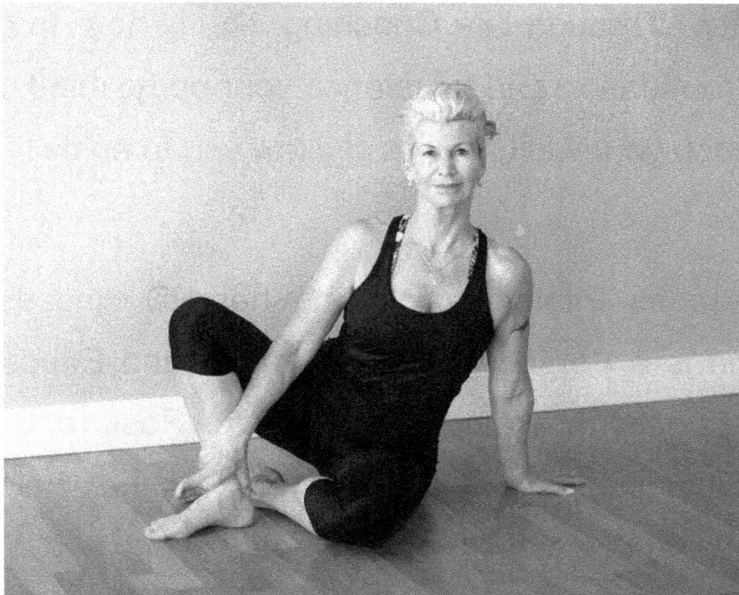

An Internationally recognized Yoga Instructor, best-selling author, Entrepreneur, Life Coach, a highly accomplished National Fitness Presenter, and a student of the Mind, Body & Spirit theory, Rhona Parsons "lights up" guiding and instructing others to live their best life through fitness, health, and wellness.

Rhona has followed her love and passion for helping others by developing and teaching fitness and yoga programs for over 21 years. She enjoys a successful fitness and wellness career leading dynamic personal and group fitness classes, core-based Yoga Vinyasa classes as well as instructor-training workshops. Many fitness and yoga instructors have been mentored by Rhona throughout BC and Alberta by attending her own creative

Continuing Education approved workshops. Currently, she is teaching her signature course, Antaraka Yoga/Pyfusion, to instructors across Canada.

With enthusiasm and passion for helping others, Rhona's professional goals are to share her extensive knowledge with you, supporting and motivating you along your journey to better health and longevity. Through Life Coaching, she is here to help you build a strong foundation and to balance your body, mind, and spirit that will enhance your wellbeing, and allow you to enjoy life to its fullest.

Locally, Rhona teaches Pilates, Yoga and her PD classes at various studios and is a Personal Fitness Trainer and Educator. She specializes in Functional Training that includes Posture, Core, Balance, Pelvic Floor Fitness, and Strength Training; helping people with balance and instability. As a body, mind and spirit innovator, Rhona leads annual sold-out weekly Yoga Retreats in Mexico where her clients are treated to five-star luxury while they relax, restore, renew and recharge their body, mind, and spirit.

Rhona is a caring, passionate person who loves her work. She is a unique and focused individual and continuously upgrades her skills to be able to teach and help others. Incredible focus and dedication to her beliefs are always evident, and her ability to motivate clients through her vast knowledge is truly inspiring. Full of boundless energy, fun, and a caring, loving individual, Rhona is a clear, concise, and methodical instructor who motivates others to take care of themselves and be kind to each other.

Rhona is a mother of 3 beautiful daughters, NanaRho to 8 incredible grandchildren, and is married to the love of her life, her firefighter hubby, Brian. She lives her truth by balancing her dedication to her career and clients, and her devotion to her family and their wellbeing.

Rhona offers a free 15-minute consultation to everyone who is looking for a new change in his/her life through fitness, health, and wellness. She can be reached by:

Website: www.rhonaparsons.com/book-online

Email: rhona@rhonaparsons.com

Linked In: linkedin.com/in/rhona-parsons-3b534784

Facebook: BodyWorks with Rhona Parsons, The Balance Coach

SOURCES

1. Jose Janssen, Armstrong, BC

2. Laura Wilson, Vernon, BC

3. McConnell, Marian Mugs., *Letters from the Yoga Masters,* North Atlantic Books

4. Parkinson Society British Columbia. www.parkinson.bc.ca/

5. Parkinson's UK. www.parkinsons.org.uk

6. O'Brien, Eimear, Brand Communications., World Parkinson's Disease Day. www. ucb.com

7. Mayfield Brain & Spine., www.mayfieldclinic.com/pe-pd.htm

8. Yoga from The Heart., Sarasota, Florida www.yogafromtheheart.com

9. PWR! Parkinson's Wellness Recovery, Tucson, Arizona www.pwr4life.org

www.ingramcontent.com/pod-product-compliance
Lightning Source LLC
Chambersburg PA
CBHW080207300326

41934CB00038B/3393